www.wadsworth.com

wadsworth.com is the World Wide Web site for Wadsworth and is your direct source to dozens of online resources.

At *wadsworth.com* you can find out about supplements, demonstration software, and student resources. You can also send email to many of our authors and preview new publications and exciting new technologies.

wadsworth.com
Changing the way the world learns®

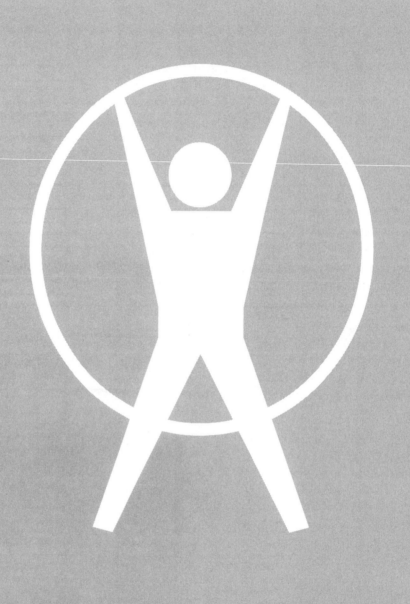

Aerobics Today

Second ▼ Edition

Carole Casten
California State University, Dominguez Hills

Peg Jordan
Health & Lifestyle, Inc.

Series Editor
Bob O'Connor

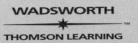

WADSWORTH
THOMSON LEARNING

Australia • Canada • Mexico • Singapore • Spain • United Kingdom • United States

WADSWORTH
THOMSON LEARNING

Publisher: Peter Marshall
Associate Editor: April Lemons
Assistant Editor: John Boyd
Editorial Assistant: Andrea Kesterke
Marketing Manager: Joanne Terhaar
Marketing Assistant: Justine Ferguson
Advertising Project Manager: Brian Chaffee
Project Manager: Sandra Craig

Print/Media Buyer: Tandra Jorgensen
Permissions Editor: Stephanie Keough-Hedges
Production and Composition: Carlisle Publishers Services
Text and Cover Designer: Harry Voigt
Copy Editor: Chris Feldman
Cover Image: Simon Wilkinson/The Image Bank, 2001
Printer: Phoenix Color/Book Technology Park

Printed in the United States of America
1 2 3 4 5 6 7 05 04 03 02 01

For permission to use material from this text, contact us by
Web: http://www.thomsonrights.com
Fax: 1-800-730-2215
Phone: 1-800-730-2214

Library of Congress Cataloging-in-Publication Data
Casten, Carole M. Sokolow.
    Aerobics today / Carole Casten, Peg Jordan. — 2nd ed.
        p. cm. — (Wadsworth's physical education series)
    Includes index.
    ISBN 0-534-35833-0
    1. Aerobic exercises. I. Jordan, Peg. II. Title. III. Series.
RA781.15 .C37 2001
613.7'15—dc21   2001045344

Wadsworth/Thomson Learning
10 Davis Drive
Belmont, CA 94002-3098
USA

For more information about our products, contact us:
Thomson Learning Academic Resource Center
1-800-423-0563
http://www.wadsworth.com

International Headquarters
Thomson Learning
International Division
290 Harbor Drive, 2nd Floor
Stamford, CT 06902-7477
USA

UK/Europe/Middle East/South Africa
Thomson Learning
Berkshire House
168-173 High Holborn
London WC1V 7AA
United Kingdom

Asia
Thomson Learning
60 Albert Street, #15-01
Albert Complex
Singapore 189969

Canada
Nelson Thomson Learning
1120 Birchmount Road
Toronto, Ontario M1K 5G4
Canada

Dedication

I would like to dedicate this book to my daughter, Kimberly, my husband, Rich, and my mother. Without their support and patience, this book would not have been possible. My husband, Rich, deserves special thanks for all of his outstanding computer skills and assistance. Without his help, completing this project would have been much more difficult. I want to thank my co-author, Peg, for her friendship, good humor, and good writing. My thanks also goes to Bob O'Connor for initially offering the opportunity to write this textbook, and my colleague, John Johnson, for his confidence in my writing. Special thanks are also given to the models used throughout the textbook.

Carole Casten, Ph.D.

The information I've shared in this book has been gathered from the innovative thinking and creations of Dr. Kenneth Cooper, Jacki Sorensen, and Marti Steele West. I dedicate this book to them, and their boundless aerobic energy. I would like to acknowledge Nancy Gillette and Linda Shelton for their contributions to injury prevention and safe instruction, and to Bonnie Rote for her work in prenatal exercise. My thanks go to my co-author, Carole Casten, for her skilled teaching expertise and her lighthearted, positive attitude that overcame each obstacle to completing this project with me.

Peg Jordan, R.N.

About the Authors

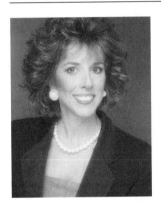

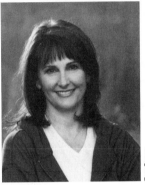

Tom Graves

Carole Casten

Carole Casten, Ph.D., is a Professor of Physical Education and Dance at California State University, Dominguez Hills, and she served as department chair for five years. She introduced dance exercise classes to the university curriculum, and she was the founding Coordinator of Dance at the university. Dr. Casten is a well-known presenter at professional conferences throughout the United States. She has held numerous offices in professional organizations and has published articles and three text-books, including *Aqua Aerobics Today.* She has also been interviewed on national radio and television as an authority in the field of dance and exercise and has served as a consultant to the California Governor's Council on Physical Fitness and Sports.

Peg Jordan

Peg Jordan, R.N., M.A., is an editor and founder of AFAA's *American Fitness* mag-azine, an international health journalist, a medical anthropologist, and the author of five books. She serves on the California Governor's Council on Physical Fitness and Sports and is a member of the honorary society National Fitness Leaders Association. Her award-winning column is featured at iVillage, allhealth, MyPotential.com, and in numerous publications. As presi-dent of Health & Lifestyle, Inc., Ms. Jordan delivers keynote speeches and presentations to audiences worldwide.

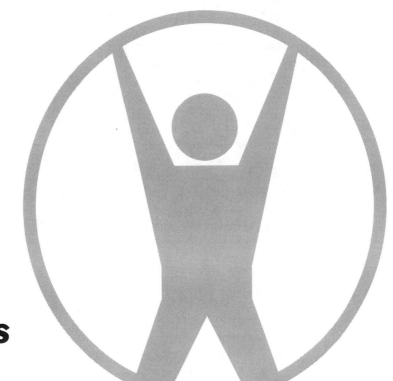

Contents

Preface   xv

1 Introduction   1
Who Created Aerobics?   2
What is Aerobics?   2
What Can You Expect to Gain from Aerobics?   4
How Much Exercise Do I Need to Be Fit?   4
Exercising for Increased Aerobic Fitness   5
Summary   5

2 Components of Fitness and Exercise   6
Components of Fitness   7
   Cardiovascular Efficiency and Endurance   8
   Muscular Strength   8
   Muscular Endurance   8
   Flexibility   8
   Body Composition   8
Your Heart   9
   Resting Heart Rate   9
   Taking The Pulse   9
   Target Heart Rate   10
Checklist for Taking Your Pulse   10
   The Karvonen Method   11
   The American College of Sports Medicine Method   11
   Recovery Heart Rate   12
   Monitoring Your Heart Rate   12
Frequency of Exercise   12
Intensity of Exercise   12
Duration of Exercise   13
Lifestyles and the Development of Cardiovascular Disease   13
Coronary Heart Disease   14
Who Gets Cardiovascular Diseases?   14
Major Risk Factors   14

Smoking 14
Excess Body Weight 14
Ideal Body Weight 14
Determining Your BMI 15
Waist Circumference 16
Calorie/Weight Chart 16
High Blood Pressure 16
High Blood Cholesterol 17
Having Your Cholesterol Checked 17
Total Blood Cholesterol 17
High-Density Lipoprotein 17
Low-Density Lipoprotein 17
Other Important Risk Factors 18
Physical Inactivity 18
Diabetes 18
Stress 18
Alcohol 18
Preventing Heart Disease 19
Summary 19

3 Committing Yourself to a Workout 20
Benefits of an Aerobic Exercise Class 21
Components of a Good Class 21
Warm-Up and Stretching 21
Checklist for Your First Aerobics Class 22
Cardiovascular/Aerobics Work 22
Checklist for Warm-Up 23
Strengthening and Toning Work 23
Cool-Down and Flexibility 23
Frequency of Workouts 23
How Long Before Results Are Apparent? 24
What to Wear to Class 24
Selecting Shoes 24
Summary 25

4 Motivation 26
Negative Motivation 27
Positive Motivation 27
Inner-Directed verses Outer-Directed 28
Why You Keep Going 28
Checklist for Mental Benefits of Aerobics 29
Setting Personal Goals 29
Following the Goals with Action 29
Checklist for Personal Goal Setting 30
Visualization 30
Checklist for Mental Imagery 31
Additional Tips to Keep you Motivated 31
Summary 31

5 Assessing Your Fitness Level 32
What Condition Are You In Now? 33
Assessing Your Personal Measurements 33
Testing Your Aerobic Capacity 34
3-Minute Step Test (Aerobic Assessment) 34
Testing Your General Flexibility 36
Student Health History 37
Summary 38
Checklist: Semester Progress Chart 39

6 Your Personal Workout   40
Your Pre-Class Warm-Up   41
Stretches and Isolations   41
   Head Isolations   41
   Shoulder Circles   42
   Rib Isolations   42
   Rib Circles   42
   Hip Isolations   42
   Hip Circles   42
   Deep Lunge   43
   Side Lunge   43
   Hamstring Stretch   43
   Quadriceps Stretch   44
   Calf Stretches   44
   Ankle Circles   44
   Ankle Raises   44
   Heel Walking   45
   Sitting Straddle Side Stretch   45
   Sitting Straddle Forward Stretch   45
Strengthening Exercises   45
   Push-Ups   45
   Reverse Push-Ups   46
   Abdominal Curl-Ups   46
   Donkey Leg Lifts   48
   Straight Leg Lifts   48
   Side Leg Lifts   48
   Bent Side Leg Lifts   49
Pelvic Lifts/Buttocks Exercise   50
Summary   50
Checklist for Your Personal Workout   51

7 Nutrition   52
Basic Nutrition Guidelines   53
Keep Variety in Your Diet   53
   Carbohydrates   53
   Fiber   53
   Proteins   53
Checklist for Calories Contained in Four Food Groups   54
   Fats   54
   Water and Hydration   54
   Vitamins and Minerals   54
   Weight Control   55
Checklist for Calculating Desirable Body Weight   56
   Body Composition   56
   Weight Loss   56
Summary   57

8 Injury Prevention   59
Prevention of Injury   60
Pain versus Exercise Discomfort   60
Treatment for Routine Injuries   60
Checklist for Treating Injuries   60
Overuse Injuries   61
   Plantar Fasciitis   61
   Achilles' Tendonitis   61
   Shin Splints   61
   Stress Reactions and Stress Fractures   61
   Knee Injuries   61

Common Causes of Aerobics Injuries   62
   Training Errors   62
   Anatomical Problems   62
   Improper Footwear   62
   Training Surfaces   62
   Program Imbalance   62
   Use of Low Weights   62
   Improper Body Alignment   63
   Muscle Imbalance   63
   Nonballistic Stretching   63
Exercises to Avoid   63
Heat and Humidity   67
Exercise-Induced Asthma   68
Exercise Intolerance   68
Cardiac Risk Factors   69
Summary   69

9   Low-Impact Aerobics   70
Definition   71
Impact and Injuries   71
Protecting the Knees   72
Low-Back Precautions   72
The Question of Weights   72
Checklist for Knee Protection   72
When Not to Use Weights   73
Low-Impact versus Low-Intensity   73
Aqua Aerobics Exercise   73
Body Sculpting   74
Other Low-Impact Alternatives   74
Benefits   74
Summary   75

10   Pregnancy and Aerobic Dance Exercise   76
Value   77
Special Precautions   77
   Medical Clearance   77
   Fluids   77
   Warning Signs that Indicate the Need to Stop Exercising   77
Modifications to an Aerobic Exercise Program   77
   Warm-Up   77
   Cardiovascular Work   78
   Floor Work   78
   Cool-Down Stretches   79
Special Exercises   80
   Low-Impact Movement   80
   Kegel Exercises   80
   Standing Work   80
Controversial Exercises   81
Exercises to Avoid   81
   High Knee Lifts   81
   Quick Lateral Movements   81
   High-Impact Jumping and Jarring   81
   Weights   81
   Traditional Rejects   81
   Prone Position   81
Summary   81

11 Selecting a Class   83
What to Look for in a Good Instructor   84
Characteristics of a Good Instructor   84
The Aerobic Dance Exercise Class   84
Checklist for Selecting a Facility   85
Selecting a Facility   85
Summary   86

12 A Guide to Buying Media for Personal Use   87
Selecting a Videotape   88
Evaluating a Videotape   88
Purchasing a Videotape   88
Selecting Music to Create Your Own Routines   88
Checklist for Videotape Evaluation   89
Summary   89

13 Being Creative: Choreographing Your Own Routines   90
Creating Your Dance Exercise Routine   91
Simple 8-Count Phrases of Movement   91
Summary   98

14 Becoming an Instructor   99
Where to Study to Become an Instructor   100
Checklist: Do I Want to Become an Instructor?   101
Summary   101
Self-Test   101

Glossary   103
Index   107

Preface

Aerobics Today is designed to assist the student of aerobic exercise in learning the basics of the activity. Additionally, this textbook offers the student the opportunity to develop and choreograph his or her own routines for fitness activity. The textbook illustrates the benefits of aerobic dance exercise for all fitness levels of involvement: from beginner to instructor, with a focus on understanding the basics. Careful attention has been given to laying the foundation for a safe and successful aerobic routine. Additionally, the authors have provided pertinent information regarding pregnancy and exercise, the mental aspect of the sport, and information for would-be instructors.

The featured photographs clearly demonstrate how to properly perform the exercises described in the book. These exercises have been found to be physically sound by exercise physiologists and recognized by certifying agencies.

The authors hope that *Aerobics Today* will be a useful tool as you make aerobic exercise a valuable part of your life.

To a healthy life!

Acknowledgments

The development of this text could not have progressed without the good advice and timely responses of the staff at Wadsworth and the textbook reviewers, or by the generosity of the models. Thank you to all involved!

Reviewers

Lois Butcher
Temple University

Felicia Cavallini
Rice College

Rhonda Kenny
East Carolina University

Tina Procacini
Mesa Community College

Lisa Tremblay
Lorain County Community College

Susan Whitlock
Kennesaw State University

Models

Melissa A. Acosta	Cho Jae Hoon
Wendy Bogdanovich	Anna Rubin
Rachelle Beyer	Wilma Uy
Debra L. Bruno	Ronica Williams
Dinah Gentry	Grace DaCanay
Cedric Gilmore	Kimbie Casten
Steve Hindman	Bao Hoang

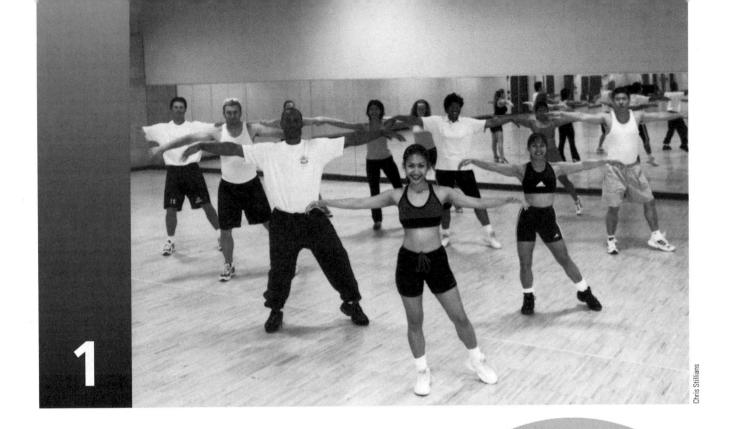

Chris Stillians

Introduction

Outline

Who Created Aerobics?

What Is Aerobics?

What Can You Expect to Gain
from Aerobics?

How Much Exercise Do I Need to
Be Fit?

Exercising for Increased Aerobic
Fitness

Summary

Aerobics is a popular form of exercise that incorporates a variety of movements performed to motivating music. Its purpose is to provide an enjoyable form of fitness development or exercise. More than 20 million people participate in aerobics annually. In fact, according to H. R. Ritchie, noted aerobics instructor, it is ranked as the sixth most popular activity in the nation.

Who Created Aerobics?

Aerobic dance was originally created in 1969 by Jacki Sorensen, a former dancer who believed in dance exercise as a beneficial form of achieving fitness. Dancercise, Jazzercise, and what is now called aerobics are variations of her original work. Although each variation is slightly different, the basic formula for an aerobics class is the same: warm-up, cardiovascular work (aerobic exercise), specific muscular strength and flexibility exercises, endurance work, and cool down.

What Is Aerobics?

The scientific definition for aerobic exercise is exercise that utilizes oxygen for a sustained activity of 2 minutes or longer. Today, aerobics refers to dance and locomotor (traveling) movements that combine in a way to force the body to utilize oxygen for a sustained period of time.

Many people who find it unpleasant or boring to jog, bicycle, swim, or jump rope find it enjoyable to move rhythmically to music. Whatever you prefer, it is important to select a fitness activity or combination of activities that you enjoy so that you will stick with it. Gaining and maintaining fitness is a lifetime commitment.

Other popular activities in which people participate for aerobic workouts include Kick Boxing, Spinning classes, Step Aerobics classes and Pilates classes. Kick Boxing uses movements that model an athletic workout for a boxer and locomotor aerobic movements used in a typical aerobics class. This workout offers the student another method in which to become fit. Spinning classes utilize a stationary bicycle, an instructor, and a room equipped with a sound system, atmospheric lights, and sometimes a video projector and screen. The participant is led through a cycling workout in which the lights, music, and the instructor create images of where the participant can imagine he or she is cycling. Additionally, the instructor directs the intensity of the workout based on the imaginary terrain through which they are cycling. Some fitness facilities utilize video projectors to guide the participant through an additional element of the workout to give the stationary bicycling experience a little more realistic feeling.

Step Aerobics classes utilize a platform designed for stability while the participant steps up from the floor to the step and back down to the floor. A variety of intricate steps, hops, slides, and turns are used to make the workout fun, varied, and challenging. Each step is assigned a name. The instructor leads the class through the workout by calling out the names of the steps, often in combination, that the class executes. The workout is performed to music similar to that used in Low-Impact Aerobics classes.

Another popular type of workout class is Body Sculpting. In this class, a body warm-up, usually modeled after traditional aerobics movements, is done, followed by stationary weight training. The weight training is sometimes alternated with a short period of aerobic exercise activity. This class has become popular because it combines aerobics and weight training in one class period.

Pilates is another type of exercise people are currently finding popular. It is a form of exercise designed to emphasize body alignment and correct breathing techniques while enhancing the two "powerhouses" in the body. The "powerhouses" are the lower abdominal muscles and the mid-back and part of the shoulders muscles. Pilates exercises work to alter patterns of movement through a change in neurological activity by using proprioception as a tool to perceive the sensation of body movements. In this form of exercise, musculo-skeletal alignment for performance is stressed.

Joseph H. Pilates developed and taught the Pilates form of exercise in the

Cycle aerobics: "spinning"

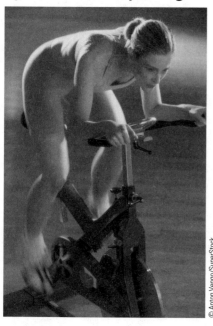

Kick boxing class

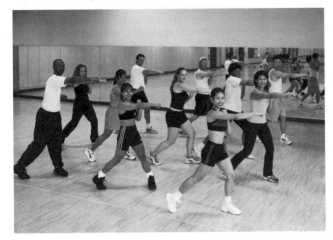

Step aerobics class

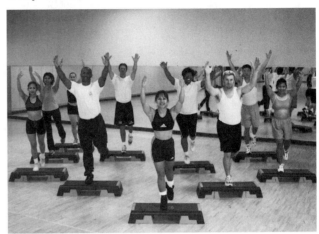

Body sculpting class

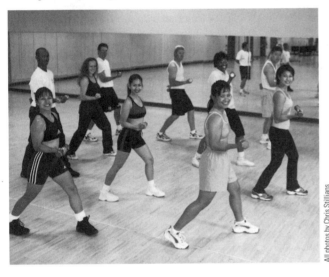

All photos by Chris Stillians

years 1916–1968 in New York. Current practitioners have taken his findings a step further by integrating body-mind energetics, as well as the bodyworks and fitness developed by Mr. Pilates, into a holistic approach of body conditioning. Pilates instructors are trying to help students develop an acute sense of body and postural awareness. While Pilates offers a vigorous muscular workout, it is not typically considered an aerobics workout.

Pilates classes can be taught in a group class setting on mats or individually. In the individual setting, the instructor often utilizes specialized equipment with spring resistance, simulating normal muscle physiology to increase strength, flexibility, coordination, and

vertebral articulation in a dynamic and functional balanced progression.

People of all ages can use Pilates for their general fitness or cross training with other sports, dance, and exercise-forms to supplement their fitness workouts.

Note: Pilates® Exercise has no affiliation with any other organization of the same name. Pilates, owned by Manuela P. Thomi and Marc Hamburger is a registered Trademark (Reg. 426605) in Switzerland.

Core Board Training is another new type of workout. Alex McKechnie, a physical therapist and consultant to a variety of professional sports teams, invented the Core Board. Mr. McKechnie needed a rehabilitation tool to get his athletes back to their games more quickly, so he built one. The Core Board enables a participant to practice the unbalanced feeling athletes experience when participating in a sport. The movements practiced in a Core board class help train the body to prevent injuries from occurring when the desired action or movement intended does not go as planned. Core board classes provide a total body workout of strength, agility, quickness, and aerobic activities.

What Can You Expect to Gain from Aerobics?

People take aerobic exercise classes for many reasons. Some people like to dance and feel this is a good way to move to music, perform locomotor dance steps, exercise, and have fun all at the same time. Others take aerobic exercise classes because they prefer not to exercise outdoors, and these forms of exercise are usually performed indoors. Still others participate in aerobics because their friends are doing it or because the class offers them the opportunity to meet new people with similar interests.

How Much Exercise Do I Need to Be Fit?

"How much exercise do I need to be fit?" is a frequently asked question. In the past, professionals have looked upon fitness as a maximum level of cardiovascular endurance and efficiency. It required increasing the heart rate significantly for 30 minutes a day in aerobic endurance activities, based on the aerobic theories of Dr. Kenneth Cooper that were advanced at Stanford University, then adopted by the American College of Sports Medicine. This standard required that one start with a maximum heart rate of 220 beats per minute, then adjust it by subtracting his or her age to get the maximum heart rate. Participants were then advised to exercise at a rate of 65 to 85 percent of that age-adjusted heart rate for 20 to 30 minutes at least three or four times per week. Some have now extended the range from 60 to 90 percent of one's maximum heart rate. The higher

number is for the better-conditioned participant.

In the 1990s, Dr. Steven Blair, the primary epidemiologist at Dr. Cooper's Aerobic Research Institute in Dallas, Texas developed a new theory. Based on his analysis of 25,000 men who were examined at the institute, he suggested that exercising for a half hour a day is enough to extend one's life. That exercise does not have to be done all at one time. The participant can walk 5 minutes in the morning, garden for 15 minutes later in the day, climb stairs for 30 seconds, then walk for 10 minutes later in the day. This accumulated exercise indicated an increase in one's life span and was more easily obtainable. The regular exercise will even reduce the risks of smoking somewhat.[1] Dr. Blair is the former president of the American College of Sports Medicine and is perhaps the world's most respected authority in the area of fitness and death risk. The Surgeon General's report, *Healthy People 2010,* also supports the theory of accumulating 30 minutes of any combined types of exercise per day.

While 30 minutes of low-level exercises a day will increase one's life span, a more vigorous exercise program appears to reduce the risk of death and increase the health benefits even more. Therefore, the American College of Sports Medicine has been re-evaluating its position. This could be the reason that both Dr. Cooper and Dr. Blair run several miles nearly every day. It seems that for maximum fitness the premise of 30 minutes a day with a significant rise in pulse rate still seems ideal—if not minimal. Of course, if you choose to exercise for more than 30 minutes per day you will burn more calories, which contributes to weight loss. It would also reduce the risk of some types of diabetes. There can also be an additional reduction of risk for heart disease. However, the wear and tear on the joints from daily aerobics or running might be a negative risk factor. More than half an

---

[1](Blair, S. N. et al. "Influences of cardiorespiratory fitness and other precursors on cardiovascular disease and all-cause mortality in men and women." *Journal of the American Medical Association 276:*205–210, 1996).

hour of exercise a day should only be done if it is enjoyable and does not cause any physical pain.

An American study[2] suggests burning a weekly output of 2,000 calories in exercise in order to achieve a minimal level of fitness. This would require 5 hours of exercise per week with an expenditure of 8 calories per minute.

Exercising for Increased Aerobic Fitness

Effective aerobic exercise, according to the American College of Sports Medicine (ACSM), requires that aerobic exercise be performed three to five times per week for 20 to 60 minutes each session at an intensity of 60 to 90 percent of the maximum heart rate, or 50 to 85 percent of the maximal oxygen consumption. (In addition, ACSM recommends the inclusion of a strength-training program for overall health benefits.)

Whatever your reason for participating in aerobics classes, you can expect the following results if you attend a class three to five times a week for at least 8 weeks. Though scientific research does not support all the following claims, people who regularly participate in aerobic dance exercise report that by following a regular exercise regime you will:

■ have more energy

■ feel better about yourself

■ change your body composition by losing fat and increasing your lean body mass

■ look more toned

■ increase your strength and flexibility

■ increase your endurance

■ meet new people and make new friends

---

[2](Paffenbarger, R. S. et al. "Some interrelationships of physical activity, physiological fitness, health and longevity." In Bouchard, C. et al. *Physical Activity in Fitness and Health.* pp. 119–133. Champaign, IL. Human Kinetics, 1993.)

■ improve your digestion

■ improve the quality of your sleep

■ reduce your stress and the byproducts of stress

■ reduce your resting heart rate

■ improve your lung capacity

■ reduce the risk of cardiovascular disease

■ invoke a sense of discipline into your daily regimen

■ invoke a sense of well-being into your daily life

Summary

1. Jacki Sorensen developed aerobic dance exercise in 1969.

2. The format of aerobics classes has changed over the years, as has its popularity. A larger variety of movements are now used in aerobics classes, such as Kick Boxing, Spinning, Step Aerobics, and High-Low Impact Aerobics. Today, more than 20 million people participate regularly in aerobic dance exercise.

3. Aerobic exercise is defined as movements combined in such a way as to cause the body to utilize oxygen for a sustained period of time.

4. To see results, it is important to participate in aerobic exercise for at least 8 weeks, three to five times per week, 20 to 60 minutes per session.

5. The reasons people participate in aerobics instead of other forms of exercise vary greatly, from simply enjoying aerobics to being able to exercise with friends.

6. The benefits of participating in aerobic exercise include feeling better, looking better, losing weight, gaining muscle tone, reducing the resting heart rate, increasing lung capacity, gaining energy, improving the immune system, and improving overall body fitness.

7. While the accumulation of 30 minutes a day of a variety of low-level exercises will increase one's life span, it appears that a more vigorous exercise program will reduce the risk of death and increase the health benefits even more.

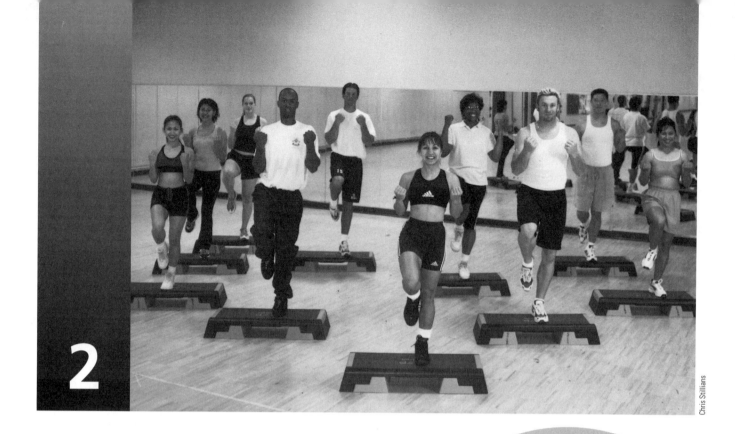

Chris Stillians

Components of Fitness and Exercise

Outline

Components of Fitness
  Cardiovascular Efficiency and
    Endurance
  Muscular Strength
  Muscular Endurance
  Flexibility
  Body Composition
Your Heart
  Resting Heart Rate
  Taking the Pulse
Checklist for Taking Your Pulse
  Target Heart Rate
    The Karvonen Method
    The American College of
      Sports Medicine Method
  Recovery Heart Rate
  Monitoring Your Heart Rate
Frequency of Exercise
Intensity of Exercise

Duration of Exercise
Lifestyles and the Development
    of Cardiovascular Disease
Coronary Heart Disease
Who Gets Cardiovascular
    Diseases?
Major Risk Factors
  Smoking
  Excess Body Weight
  High Blood Pressure
  High Blood Cholesterol
Other Important Risk Factors
  Physical Inactivity
  Diabetes
  Stress
  Alcohol
Preventing Heart Disease
Summary

The benefits of aerobic exercise are numerous. Research has firmly established that regular, vigorous exercise is beneficial to the human body. One major benefit is that, after aerobically exercising, an individual feels "good" and exhilarated. Another benefit of aerobic exercise is a reduction of stress and tension in the body. Other benefits of regular exercise include an increased overall fitness level and a better-toned physique. The well-conditioned person is also able to ward off infectious diseases and cancers better than the poorly conditioned person, because the immune system is strengthened through exercising on a regular basis. Additionally, coronary risk is lowered by increasing the beneficial type of cholesterol, high-density lipoproteins (HDLs), and reducing the ratio of total cholesterol to HDL. The liver manufactures about 75 percent of your body's cholesterol. The liver changes the cholesterol into low-density lipoproteins (LDLs) and triglycerides. The LDLs and triglycerides enter the bloodstream and are deposited into various tissues. Excess LDL-cholesterol is deposited along arterial walls. This forms the plaque that blocks the bloodstream. Any HDLs in the area remove excess cholesterol from the bloodstream.

Another benefit of aerobic exercising is that muscle fibers increase in size and perform more efficiently. Also, bones are strengthened, become more dense, and are more resistant to deterioration. Weight control is easier because aerobic exercise raises your metabolic rate, burning additional calories, increasing fat utilization, and improving digestion and elimination. Additionally, the body becomes more physically fit. The heart muscle becomes stronger and more efficient, lung capacity increases, muscles increase in strength and endurance, and the body becomes more flexible. In short, aerobic exercise offers both psychological and physiological benefits.

Athletes and physiologists of exercise have observed the mental effects of exercise. High-level performers have generally shown higher than average levels of social maturity, self-confidence, and intellectual efficiency. A study at Purdue University showed that untrained middle-aged university employees significantly improved their mental outlooks during the duration of a specially designed fitness program of calisthenics and jogging. Results of the study showed that statistically-significant positive changes had occurred. The areas of self-assurance, stability, and imagination were all greatly improved in the test subjects.

The circulation of blood to the brain during exercise aids in making one more alert. Some people have found that physical activity allows one to take out aggressions and become more relaxed in the process. When people exercise, they may be unconsciously taking out frustrations which might otherwise be directed at a boss, a teacher, or a parent.

There is a substance, called catecholamine, that is essential in several brain chemicals to help transmit messages in the brain. One of the essential precursors for this brain chemical is called tyrosine hydroxylase (TH). TH decreases with age and may be a factor in age-related mental changes and problems. The Geriatric Research, Education, and Clinical Center of the Department of Veterans Affairs Medical Center in Gainesville, Florida has done a study with rats which showed that exercise reduced the loss of TH. If further study proves this to be true with humans, we may have another mental benefit of endurance exercises.[1]

Components of Fitness

An individual is considered to be physically fit when these five components of fitness are developed and balanced:

1. cardiovascular efficiency and endurance

2. muscular strength

3. muscular endurance

4. flexibility

5. body composition

---

[1] (Tumer N, LaRochelle JS, Yurekli M. "Exercise training reverses the age-related decline in tyrosine hydroxylase expression in rat hypothalamus," *J Gerontol A Biol Sci Med Sci* 1997 Sep; 52(5): pp. 255–259)

It is important that you understand these five components so that you know what is necessary to keep your body in top shape inside and outside.

Cardiovascular Efficiency and Endurance

Cardiovascular efficiency and endurance refers to the body's ability to deliver oxygen to all of its vital organs. The efficiency of the heart and respiratory system determines how well the body provides oxygen to its vital organs during exercise and while at rest. The cardiovascular system consists of the heart, lungs, and blood vessels. At all times, but particularly during the stress of exercise, the cardiovascular system must be able to transport oxygen efficiently to provide the needed energy to the heart, lungs, and working muscles. An efficient cardiovascular system is essential to a high level of physical fitness. Exercise increases the strength of the heart, which increases its ability to pump blood most efficiently throughout the body.

Cardiovascular endurance, or aerobic fitness, is the ability of the heart and respiratory system to deliver blood, and therefore oxygen, to the working muscles during prolonged exercise.

Muscular Strength

Muscular strength is the amount of force produced when a muscle group contracts and moves a resistance one time. Strength is essential for a variety of everyday activities, such as lifting and moving objects; opening doors, jars, and windows; carrying children; and walking up stairs. Muscular strength is increased when the muscle is overloaded by repetitive activities and/or when a resistance or weight is added to the muscle. (A resistance is any amount of additional weight the body moves.)

Muscular Endurance

Muscular endurance is the ability of the muscles to exert force over an extended period of time. Endurance is an important element in helping you participate in repetitive activities, such as aerobics, jogging, swimming, walking, dancing, and stair climbing.

Flexibility

Flexibility is the range of motion possible in the joints. Flexibility is necessary to maintain body mobility. The more flexible you are, the more easily you can move your limbs through their full range of motion. The more flexible your muscles are, the fewer sore muscles and joint injuries you will have. Inactivity can produce the effect of tightening or shortening the muscles, thereby yielding a greater risk of injury when the muscles are put to use or stressed even a little.

Body Composition

Body composition is the relation of body fat to lean body mass (muscle, bone, cartilage, and vital organs). To be considered lean, women must have less than 22 percent of their weight in fat, and men must have less than 15 percent.

We are all born with a genetically determined body type. There are three kinds of body types or somatotypes: mesomorph, endomorph, and ectomorph. The mesomorph is characterized as having a predominance of muscle and bone and is often labeled "very muscular-looking." Mesomorphic body types perform best in activities requiring strength, speed, and agility. The endomorph is a soft and round-looking individual with an excess of adipose or fatty tissue. Endomorphic body types have difficulty performing aerobic and skill-oriented activities. Ectomorphic body types are very thin and lean. These people do well in endurance activities, such as aerobics, but may have difficulty in activities requiring strength.

Don't fret if you don't fit into one body-type classification. Very few people are classified as being exclusively one somatotype. Usually a person is a combination of types (such as the mesomorphic endomorph, who appears muscular yet has a rounded look). The importance of knowing this information is to realize that we are all different. Your goal must be personal. Your objective should be to

Somatotypes

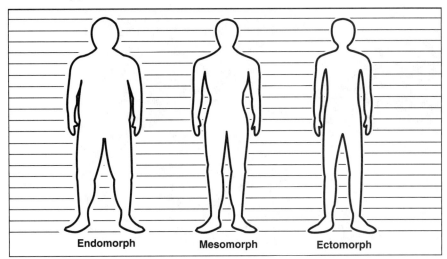

| Endomorph | Mesomorph | Ectomorph |

be the best you can with the body you inherited.

It is important to the quality of your life and health that you are at least minimally fit in each of the components of fitness. A person who is minimally physically fit has enough strength and endurance to perform daily tasks without undue fatigue and has enough energy left to enjoy leisure activities and be able to deal with an emergency situation.

Your Heart

Scientific evidence indicates that regular cardiovascular exercise strengthens the heart muscle and reduces the risk of cardiovascular problems. Through exercise overload, the heart muscle becomes more fit and is able to work more efficiently and effectively. Exercise overload occurs when the body is subjected to greater exercise stress than it is accustomed to. When you perform exercise overload in a progressive and moderate amount, you strengthen muscles. However, if exercise overload is done in a nonprogressive, uncontrolled, and excessive manner, injury might occur. The more fit the heart is, the more oxygen-carrying blood can be pumped to the body with each contraction of the heart. Thus, a fit heart does not need to work as hard or beat as frequently as a less-fit

heart. In discussing cardiovascular fitness and efficiency, you need to be aware of your resting heart rate, your target heart rate, and your recovery heart rate.

Resting Heart Rate

Resting heart rate refers to the number of times your heart beats per minute upon waking or when you have been sitting or resting for approximately 10 minutes. The best time to take your resting heart rate is when you first wake up and are still lying down. To obtain the most accurate reading, take your pulse for 60 seconds on two consecutive mornings, and then average the two numbers. A person who exercises regularly may have a lower resting heart rate than a person who is sedentary. An average resting heart rate is about 72 beats per minute. If you discover your resting heart rate has decreased after you've done a few months of regular aerobic exercise, it indicates you are increasing your level of fitness. That's a sign you would like to see.

Taking the Pulse

For most people, taking the pulse is easiest at the carotid artery. The carotid pulse is located in the groove of the neck, next to the Adam's apple. Use your first two fingers and press lightly on the carotid artery (be careful not to press too hard). You will feel your pulse.

Another place to take your pulse is at the radial artery (on the thumb side of

Taking pulse at the carotid artery

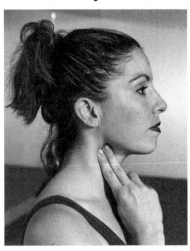

Chris Stillians

Taking pulse at the radial artery

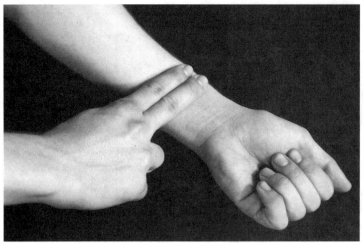

Chris Stillians

your wrist, palm up). When taking your pulse, be sure to use the first two or three fingers, not the thumb. The thumb has a pulse of its own and therefore could cause an inaccurate reading.

Target Heart Rate

Heart rate is widely accepted as a good method for measuring intensity during aerobic exercise. Exercise that raises your heart rate to a certain level and keeps it there for 20 minutes will significantly contribute to a cardiovascular fitness level improvement.

The heart rate you should maintain while aerobically exercising is called your target heart rate. Target heart rate

(THR) is the level at which you will gain the benefits of exercising your heart to improve cardiovascular fitness. There are two accepted formulas for calculating your target heart rate presented on page 11. Use both formulas, compare the two results, and then choose the level where you will work. (You may choose an average of the two results.)

First, you need to determine the intensity level at which you would like to work. A person who has been sedentary for a long time may want to begin an exercise regimen at the 60 percent level and gradually work up to 70 percent. It is generally accepted that, for most people, 70 percent is a good level at which to work. Athletes and highly fit individuals may work at 85 percent.

 Checklist for Taking Your Pulse

1. With your index and middle fingers (not your thumb) you can find your pulse in the carotid artery very easily, by:

   Placing your fingers on your Adam's apple. Gently slide your fingers toward the outside of the neck, into the natural "notch" on the side of your neck. By pressing lightly, you can feel the pulse at the carotid artery.

2. You can find your radial pulse by:

   Placing your fingers lightly on the inside of your wrist. To do this, rotate one arm in so the palm of your hand is facing you. Then place the fingers

   of the opposite hand just above your wrist on the thumb side of your arm and just inside the arm bone (the radius). You will feel the radial pulse.

3. Count the number of pulse beats for a minute. You can do this by:

   - counting your pulse for 30 seconds and multiplying by 2
   - counting your pulse for 15 seconds and multiplying by 4
   - counting your pulse for 10 seconds and multiplying by 6

   The 10-second count is preferred when you are taking your pulse during exercise.

Second, you must determine your resting heart rate. Once you determine your intensity level and your resting heart rate, proceed with the formulas listed below.

Many fitness professionals are now using a heart target rate formula developed by the Finnish physiologist Karvonen. It adds the component of using the maximum heart rate (that is, the heart reserve) to calculate your target heart rate. This formula takes into account one's resting heart rate in addition to one's maximal heart rate.

To determine your maximal oxygen consumption rate (VO_2 max), you can complete the Rockport Fitness Walking Test.[2] This test has been validated by ACSM as an acceptable fitness test. *The Rockport Fitness Walking Test is conducted as follows:*

1. Choose a windless day to conduct the test.

2. Record your weight.

3. Walk 1 mile as fast as possible.

4. Record the time to complete the 1-mile walk.

5. Immediately upon finishing the walk, record your heart rate in a 10-second interval. Multiply that number by 6 to find the beats per minute.

6. Use this number as your maximal oxygen consumption rate in the Karvonen method listed below.

Now that you have found your maximal oxygen consumption rate, you can monitor yourself to see how well your cardiorespiratory fitness program is working by occasionally repeating the above test. As your fitness level increases, your VO_2 max will increase because cardiorespiratory fitness relies on the effective delivery and use of oxygen to produce energy. You can also measure your progress by noting the changes in your resting pulse rate. As your fitness levels improve, your resting pulse rate should decrease.

The Karvonen Method

The Karvonen method of determining the target heart rate for a 20-year-old

person working at 70 percent intensity is as follows:

THR = (MHR–RHR) × .70 + RHR
where
THR = target heart rate
MHR = maximum heart rate
RHR = resting heart rate
To determine the THR in this example, calculate:
220 − age = maximum heart rate (MHR)[3]
220 − 20 = 200
200 − resting heart rate (RHR) = heart rate range
200 − 80 = 120
120 × the desired intensity of activity (70%)
120 × .70 = 84
Heart rate range + the resting heart rate = target heart rate
84 + 80 = 164 beats per minute
164 = target heart rate (THR)
Divide the target heart rate by 6 to get the number you need for a 10-second pulse count: 164 ÷ 6 = 27

The American College of Sports Medicine Method

The American College of Sports Medicine recommends a simpler formula. Subtract your age from 220, multiply by the desired intensity of your workout level, and divide the answer by 6 for a 10-second pulse estimate. It is recommended that your working target heart rate be 65 to 85 percent of your maximum heart rate.

The following example is again for a 20-year-old working at the 70 percent level:
220 − 20 = 200 maximum heart rate
200 × .7 = 140 target heart rate (THR)
140 ÷ 6 = 23 number of pulse beats in a 10-second period
To work at the desired level of intensity, this 20-year-old would consider the results of both formulas and strive for 23 to 27 pulse beats during a 10-second count.

Be careful not to work over your target heart rate for more than a few seconds. You will not get into shape any faster. Working over your target heart rate may fatigue you faster, cause you

---

[2](Kline, Porcari, Hintermeister, Freedson, Ward, McCarron, Ross, and Rippe, 1987).

[3]Note: This formula can be used to estimate your MHR if you did not complete the Rockport Fitness Walking Test.

discomfort, and even be unhealthy for you. Use common sense to check your exertion: If you are feeling extreme fatigue, you are probably overworking yourself.

Recovery Heart Rate

Your recovery heart rate is how quickly your pulse returns to normal after an aerobic workout. The more aerobically conditioned you are, the faster your heart will return to normal, or recover. Take your pulse 2 to 5 minutes after exercising. Your heart rate should be below 100 beats per minute.

Recovery Heart Rate Chart

Take your pulse 2 to 5 minutes after exercising. If you have a decrease from your target heart rate of:

60 beats per minute = super recovery rate

50 beats per minute = excellent recovery rate

40 beats per minute = good

30 beats per minute = acceptable

After several months of consistently working out aerobically, you may notice that your heart rate recovers faster and is lower than before you began your exercise regimen. Your heart rate should return to its pre-exercise level within 10 minutes after class ends. If it doesn't, you may have overexerted yourself during the aerobics portion of class. Reduce the intensity of your workout during the next class, and monitor the length of time it takes for your heart rate to return to normal.

Monitoring Your Heart Rate

Monitoring your heart rate during exercise is extremely important. Take your pulse several times during, and especially immediately following, the aerobics portion of class. When checking your heart rate during a workout, take your pulse within 5 seconds after you stop exercising aerobically because it starts to go down once you stop moving. Count your pulse for 10 seconds, and multiply by 6 to get the per-minute rate. Your instructor will most likely lead the group in monitoring the heart rate following aerobic exercise. If not, monitor your heart rate yourself.

You need to make sure you are working within your appropriate target heart rate zone. If, when checking your pulse, you discover you are working at too high a level, adjust your movements to reduce the intensity of the workout. To reduce the intensity of exercise, keep your arms lower than your heart and don't lift your legs as high as you did previously. If you find you are not working as high as your target heart rate, increase your workload by making larger movements or lifting your arms or legs higher. However, never lift your legs higher than hip level.

Frequency of Exercise

Frequency of exercise refers to how often you exercise per week. To obtain benefits from working out, you should participate in the aerobic portion of class three to five times a week for 20 to 30 minutes per session. If you exercise only once a week, your fitness level may improve minimally, and you may be sore after exercising because of the stress you have placed on unconditioned muscles. Exercising every day is not necessary either. Studies show that people who rest at least one day a week have fewer injuries than those who exercise daily. Similarly, exercising three to five times a week appears to be nearly as beneficial as exercising six or seven times a week. The body needs time to rest and recuperate so that you can avoid strained muscles and shin splints. An occasional day off is of great value in developing and maintaining fitness, both physically and psychologically.

Intensity of Exercise

Intensity of exercise refers to how hard you work when exercising. Once you have identified your target heart rate, you should continually monitor the intensity at which you are working. Working too hard is ineffective, as it can make you sore and may result in an injury. The key is to find the optimal level of intensity for your body and to meet your goals.

Duration of Exercise

Duration of exercise refers to how long you work out at one time. The duration of your exercise sessions depends on the components of fitness you are trying to develop.

You must spend time on each component of fitness you are trying to develop, as well as time on each muscle group. For each component, you must do at least 5 continuous minutes of exercise at one time. For the cardiovascular component, you must do a minimum of 20 continuous minutes of concentrated effort in your target heart rate zone. According to the American College of Sports Medicine (ACSM), aerobic exercise should be engaged in three to five times per week for 20 to 60 minutes each session, at an intensity of 60 to 90 percent of maximum heart rate or 50 to 85 percent of maximal oxygen consump-

tion. (In addition, ACSM recommends the inclusion of a strength-training program for overall health benefits.) As mentioned earlier, a 50-minute aerobic exercise class that meets three to five times per week provides you with a good duration of weekly exercise to meet most of your goals.

Lifestyles and the Development of Cardiovascular Disease

Studies show that certain attributes, habits, and styles of living have a high degree of correlation with the development of cardiovascular disease. Factors known to increase the risks of cardiovascular disease include a family history of heart disease, high blood pressure, cigarette smoking, being overweight, high levels of triglycerides and cholesterol in the blood, diabetes, stress, menopause, and physical inactivity. An analysis of your personal risk factors will guide you toward achieving a healthy lifestyle.

To perform a self-analysis of your fitness awareness, complete the following self-test.

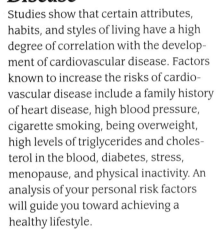

Self-Test

Answer *yes* or *no* to each question.

_____ 1. I climb stairs rather than take the elevator whenever possible.

_____ 2. I know my resting pulse rate.

_____ 3. I know my blood pressure.

_____ 4. I know that aerobic exercise at least three times a week will reduce my heart attack risk.

_____ 5. I participate in aerobic exercise at least three times per week.

_____ 6. I know my target heart rate for aerobic exercise.

_____ 7. I execute abdominal curl-ups at least three times a week.

_____ 8. I perform exercises for my lower back at least three times per week.

_____ 9. I believe that exercise will improve my mental health.

_____ 10. I know that aerobic exercise is one of the best things I can do to maintain my desired weight.

Test Evaluation

9 to 10 *yes* answers indicate that you are quite aware of your physical fitness and its importance.

7 to 8 *yes* answers indicate a fair understanding of the principles of physical fitness.

5 to 6 *yes* answers indicate that you need to improve your knowledge and behavior in the physical fitness area.

Coronary Heart Disease

Both heart disease and stroke are known as cardiovascular diseases. They are disorders of the heart and blood vessel system. Coronary heart disease is a disease of the blood vessels of the heart that causes heart attacks. A heart attack often occurs when an artery becomes blocked, preventing oxygen and nutrients from getting to the heart. A stroke occurs when not enough blood gets to the brain. In some cases, it can occur from diseases, including high blood pressure, angina (chest pain), rheumatic heart disease, and other cardiovascular diseases.

Who Gets Cardiovascular Diseases?

Some people have more "risk factors" for cardiovascular diseases than others. Risk factors are habits or genetic traits that make a person more likely to develop a disease. Genetic risk factors for heart-related problems cannot be changed, but many others can be. The four biggest risk factors for cardiovascular disease that an individual can control are: cigarette smoking, excess body weight, high blood pressure, and high blood cholesterol. Other risk factors, such as diabetes, are also conditions of which you have less control. The more risk factors you have, the more likely you are to develop cardiovascular diseases—and the more concerned you should be about protecting your heart's health.

Major Risk Factors

Smoking

If you smoke, you are two to six times more likely to suffer a heart attack than a nonsmoker, and the risk increases with the number of cigarettes you smoke each day. Smoking also boosts the risk of stroke.

Cardiovascular diseases are not the only health risks connected to smoking. People who smoke are much more likely to develop lung cancer than nonsmokers. Smokers are also more likely to develop other kinds of lung problems, including bronchitis and emphysema. Cigarette smoking is also linked with cancers of the mouth, larynx, esophagus, urinary tract, kidney, pancreas, and cervix.

Excess Body Weight

Excess body weight is linked with coronary heart disease, stroke, congestive heart failure, and death from heart-related causes. The more overweight you are, the higher your risk for heart disease.

When an individual is overweight it contributes not only to cardiovascular diseases, but also to other risk factors, including high blood pressure, high blood cholesterol, and the most common type of diabetes. Fortunately, these conditions can often be controlled with weight loss and regular physical activity.

What is a healthy weight for you? There is no exact answer. Check the "Ideal Body Weight" chart on page 15s for the weight range suggested for your height. Ranges are given because people of the same height and amounts of body fat can differ in their weights due to their bone structure and the amounts of muscle and fat on their body.

Body shape as well as weight may affect the heart's health. "Apple-shaped" individuals with extra fat at the waistline *may* have a higher risk than "pear-shaped" people with heavy hips and thighs. If your waist is nearly as large, or larger, than the size of your hips, you *may* have a higher risk for coronary heart disease.

Ideal Body Weight

The following chart shows the ideal body weight for men and women according to the U.S. Department of Agriculture (1995).

Cholesterol in blood stream

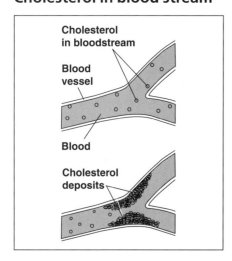

Height	Age (19–34)	Age (over 35)
5'0"	97–128	108–138
5'1"	101–132	111–143
5'2"	104–137	115–148
5'3"	107–141	119–152
5'4"	114–150	122–157
5'5"	118–155	126–162
5'6"	121–155	130–167
5'7"	121–160	134–172
5'8"	129–169	138–178
5'9"	132–174	142–183
5'10"	136–179	146–188
5'11"	140–184	151–194
6'0"	144–189	155–194
6'1"	148–195	159–205
6'2"	152–200	164–210
6'3"	156–200	168–216
6'4"	156–205	173–222
6'5"	160–211	177–228
6'6"	164–216	182–234

Body Mass Index (BMI)

The Body Mass Index (BMI), based on the U.S. government's 1998 *Clinical Guidelines on the Identification,* *Evaluation, and Treatment of Overweight and Obesity in Adults,* is a reliable system for measuring a person's body fat content. The information it provides will give you a dependable gauge of any needed weight reduction and by what degree weight loss is needed. Because the BMI is easy to understand (the higher your BMI, the greater your risk of health problems) and BMI values apply to both men and women, regardless of frame size, the BMI is a better indicator of weight variables than traditional height-weight tables.

BMI is not a reliable measurement device for:

- anyone less than 18 years old
- those with excessive muscle mass, such as highly competitive athletes and body builders
- pregnant or nursing women
- frail or sedentary elderly persons

Determining your BMI

To use the BMI table, find your height in the left-hand column and move across the row until you find your weight. The number at the top of that column will be your BMI.

Body Mass Index (BMI)	19	20	21	22	23	24	25	26	27	28	29	30	35	40
Height (feet and inches)							Weight (pounds)							
4'10"	91	96	100	105	110	115	119	124	129	134	138	143	167	191
4'11"	94	99	104	109	114	119	124	128	133	138	143	148	173	198
5'0"	97	102	107	112	118	123	128	133	138	143	148	153	179	204
5'1"	100	106	111	116	122	127	132	137	143	148	153	158	185	211
5'2"	104	109	115	120	126	131	136	142	147	153	158	164	191	218
5'3"	107	113	118	124	130	135	141	146	152	158	163	169	197	225
5'4"	110	116	122	128	134	140	145	151	157	163	169	174	204	232
5'5"	114	120	126	132	138	144	150	156	162	168	174	180	210	240
5'6"	118	124	130	136	142	148	155	161	167	173	179	186	216	247
5'7"	121	127	134	140	146	153	159	166	172	178	185	191	223	255
5'8"	125	131	138	144	151	158	164	171	177	184	190	197	230	262
5'9"	128	135	142	149	155	162	169	176	183	189	196	203	236	270
5'10"	132	139	146	153	160	167	174	181	188	195	202	207	243	278
5'11"	136	143	150	157	165	172	179	186	193	200	208	215	250	286
6'0"	140	147	154	162	169	177	184	191	199	206	213	221	258	294
6'1"	144	151	159	166	174	182	189	197	204	212	219	227	265	302
6'2"	148	155	163	171	179	186	194	202	210	218	225	233	272	311
6'3"	152	160	168	176	184	192	200	208	216	224	232	240	279	319
6'4"	156	164	172	180	189	197	205	213	221	230	238	246	287	328

You can also calculate your BMI through this formula: Multiply your weight (in pounds) by 704.5; multiply your height (in inches) by your height (in inches). Divide the first result by the second.

Example:

If you're 5'5" and weigh 140 pounds:

$140 \times 704.5 = 98,630$

$65 \times 65 = 4,225$

$98,630$ divided by $4,225 = 23$

Thus, your BMI is 23.

Once you have determined your BMI, you can reference the chart below to identify your BMI classification. If you fall within any of the categories above "Healthy Weight," your body fat level indicates that you may be suffering from obesity or an overweight condition. Weight loss to alleviate this condition is recommended for improved health.

Category	BMI
Underweight	< 18.5
Normal	18.5–24.9
Overweight	25.0–29.9
Obese (type I)	30.0–34.9
Obese (type II)	35.0–39.9
Extremely Obese	>= 40

Waist Circumference

Another important consideration in determining "fatness" is waist size. The presence of excess fat in the abdomen, out of proportion to total body fat, is an independent predictor of obesity-related risk factors and mortality. Waist circumference provides a clinically acceptable measurement for assessing one's abdominal fat content. In fact, according to the government study referenced above, simple waist circumference is a better measure than more complicated measurements, such as hip-to-waist ratio. Waist measurements greater than 40 inches for men and 35 inches for women are an indication of greater health risks.

Calorie/Weight Chart

The following chart details the number of calories you should consume to maintain a specific weight. To determine your ideal caloric intake, find your weight and move across to your age category. This is the number of calories you should consume each day to maintain that weight.

If you are not currently at your ideal weight and have a specific goal weight in mind, you can use this chart to determine how many calories you should eat to gradually achieve your desired weight. By consuming the calories for your desired weight category, your body will slowly adjust to your calorie intake and eventually reach your desired weight.

High Blood Pressure

High blood pressure, also known as hypertension, is another major risk factor for coronary heart disease and the most important risk factor for stroke. Even slightly high levels can increase your risk. High blood pressure also boosts the chances of developing kidney disease.

Women Daily Maintenance Calories*				Men Daily Maintenance Calories*			
Desirable Weight	18-35 Years	35-55 Years	55-75 Years	Desirable Weight	18-35 Years	35-55 Years	55-75 Years
99	1,700	1,500	1,300	110	2,200	1,950	1,650
110	1,850	1,650	1,400	121	2,400	2,150	1,850
121	2,000	1,750	1,550	132	2,550	2,300	1,950
128	2,100	1,900	1,600	143	2,700	2,400	2,050
132	2,150	1,950	1,650	154	2,900	2,600	2,200
143	2,300	2,050	1,800	165	3,100	2,800	2,400
154	2,400	2,150	1,850	176	3,250	2,950	2,500
165	2,550	2,300	1,950	187	3,300	3,100	2,600

*Based on moderate activity. If your life is very active, add calories; if you lead a sedentary life, subtract calories. Prepared by the Food and Nutrition Board of the National Academy of Sciences, National Research Council.

Blood pressure is the amount of force exerted by the blood against the walls of the arteries. Everyone has to have some blood pressure, so that blood can get to the body's organs and muscles. Usually, blood pressure is expressed as two numbers, such as 120/80 mm Hg. Blood pressure varies through the day and in response to your activities. It is considered high when it stays above normal levels over a period of time.

High blood pressure is called the "silent killer" because most people who have it do not feel sick. Therefore, it is important to have it checked each time you see your doctor or other health professional. Since one's blood pressure changes often, your health professional should check it on several different days before deciding if your blood pressure is too high. If your blood pressure stays at 140/90 mm Hg or above, you have high blood pressure. High blood pressure can be controlled with proper treatment. If your blood pressure is not too high, you may be able to control it entirely through weight loss (if you are overweight) and regular physical activity. Some doctors recommend reducing the intake of alcohol, table salt, and sodium. (Sodium is an ingredient in salt that is found in many packaged and processed foods, baking soda, and some antacids.) If your blood pressure remains high, your doctor may prescribe medicine in addition to the lifestyle changes described above.

Blood pressure tends to increase as one ages. That means even if your blood pressure is normal now, it makes sense to take steps to prevent high blood pressure in the years to come. You will be less likely to develop high blood pressure if you are physically active, maintain a healthy weight, limit your alcohol intake, and cut down on table salt and sodium.

High Blood Cholesterol

High blood cholesterol is another very important risk factor for coronary heart disease that you can control. Blood cholesterol levels tend to rise as one ages, particularly over the age of 40. The higher your blood cholesterol level, the higher your risk of heart diseases. The body needs cholesterol to function normally, and makes enough to fill its needs. However, cholesterol is also taken into the body through the diet. Over a period of years, extra cholesterol and fat circulating in the blood settles on the inner walls of the arteries that supply blood to the heart. These deposits make the arteries narrower and narrower. As a result, less blood gets to the heart and the risk of coronary heart disease increases.

Having Your Cholesterol Checked

Having your blood cholesterol level checked is a relatively simple process. Your doctor or other health care professional will take a small sample of your blood and measure the amount of cholesterol. When you have this test for the first time, it is important to have the following measurements taken:

Total Blood Cholesterol

For all adults, a desirable level of total blood cholesterol is less than 200 mg. A level of 240 or more means you have high blood cholesterol. But even "borderline-high" levels (200-239) boost your risk of coronary heart disease.

High-Density Lipoprotein

You will also need a measurement of your level of high-density lipoprotein, or HDL, if an accurate result is available. Lipoproteins are the packages that carry cholesterol through the bloodstream. HDL is often called "good cholesterol" because it helps remove cholesterol from the blood, preventing it from piling up in the arteries. If your HDL level is less than 35, your risk of heart disease goes up. This is true even if your total cholesterol level is within a desirable range. The good news is that if your HDL level is 60 or above, you have a lower risk of developing heart disease.

Low-Density Lipoprotein

Your doctor may also want to measure your level of low-density lipoprotein, or LDL. LDL is often called "bad cholesterol" because it carries most of the cholesterol in the blood, and if the LDL level is too high, cholesterol and fat can build up in the arteries. An LDL level below 130 is desirable, while levels of 130-159 are "borderline-high." An LDL level of 160 or above means you have a high risk of developing coronary heart disease. Cutting back on foods rich in fat, especially saturated fat and cholesterol, can lower both your total and LDL cholesterol.

Weight loss for overweight persons and increased physical activity may also lower blood cholesterol levels. Losing extra weight and becoming more physically active, as well as quitting smoking, may also help boost HDL cholesterol levels.

Other Important Risk Factors

Physical Inactivity

Various studies show that physical inactivity is a risk factor for heart disease. Heart disease is almost twice as likely to develop in inactive people as in those more active. Therefore, by participating in regular physical aerobic activity you will help lower your risk of heart disease. The best exercises to strengthen your heart and lungs are aerobics, brisk walking, jogging, cycling, and swimming. To obtain an aerobic exercise benefit, maintain activity for 30 minutes, three or four times a week.

Diabetes

Diabetes, or high blood sugar, is a serious disorder that raises the risk of coronary heart disease. The risk of death from heart disease is about three times higher in people with diabetes. Diabetics are also more apt to have high blood pressure and higher blood cholesterol than those without diabetes.

Diabetes is often called a "woman's disease" because, after age 45, about twice as many women as men develop diabetes. While there is no cure for this disorder, there are steps a person can take to control it. Being overweight and growing older are linked with the development of the most common type of diabetes. Losing excess weight and increasing physical activity levels may help postpone or prevent the disease. For lasting weight loss, regularly partici-

pate in exercise and eat foods that are low in calories and fat.

Stress

You may have read about the connection between stress and heart disease. In particular, you may have read that "Type A" behavior (being aggressive, competitive, and constantly concerned about time) is linked to the development of heart disease. Although some studies have shown this connection in men, there is little evidence that "Type A" behavior in women is linked to the development of coronary heart disease.

Employment outside the home is another factor that has often been connected to women's heart disease. At this time, studies have shown little difference in the rates of coronary heart disease between women who do not work outside the home and women employed outside of the home. However, more research is needed before stress can be ruled out as a risk factor for women.

Alcohol

Several recent studies have reported that moderate drinkers, those who have one or two drinks per day of red wine, are less likely to develop heart disease than people who don't drink any alcohol. If you are a nondrinker, this is not a recommendation to start using alcohol. And certainly, if you are pregnant or have another health condition that could make alcohol use harmful, you should not drink. But if you're already a moderate drinker of red wine, you *may* be less likely to have a heart attack.

Moderation is the key. More than two drinks per day can raise blood pressure, and binge drinking can lead to stroke. People who drink heavily on a regular basis have higher rates of heart disease than either moderate drinkers or nondrinkers.

Keep in mind, too, that alcohol provides little in the way of nutrients—mostly just extra calories. So, if you are trying to control your weight, you may want to cut down on alcohol and substitute calorie-free iced tea, soda, or seltzer.

Preventing Heart Disease

You now know about the kinds of habits, health conditions, and other factors that affect your chances of developing heart disease. Just as important, you know that by taking an active role in your own heart's health, you can make lifestyle choices to improve your health.

The American Heart Association has identified a number of steps you can take to reduce the risk of heart disease and stroke.[4] When you take them together, these steps are your best chance to win the battle for a healthy heart:

- Quit smoking, if you smoke.

- Decrease high blood pressure.

- Reduce high cholesterol and triglycerides.

- Increase your physical activity levels.

- If you are a woman and have passed menopause, talk with your doctor about hormone therapies.

- Control or delay diabetes.

- Maintain healthy weight and eat a healthful diet.

- Moderate any use of alcohol.

Summary

1. Research has established that regular vigorous exercise is beneficial to the human body in many ways. The benefits include:
- An individual feels good after exercising aerobically.
- Stress and tension in the body are reduced.

- Coronary heart disease risk is lowered.
- Muscle fibers perform more efficiently.
- Bones are strengthened.
- Weight control is easier because aerobic exercise raises your metabolic rate and allows you to burn more calories.
- The heart muscle becomes stronger and more efficient.

2. The five components of fitness are:
- cardiovascular efficiency
- muscular strength
- muscular endurance
- flexibility
- body composition

3. To understand your cardiovascular fitness and efficiency, you must be aware of and know how to calculate your:
- resting heart rate
- target heart rate
- maximum heart rate
- recovery heart rate

4. You can easily take your pulse by checking the carotid or the radial artery.

5. The minimum number of times you need to exercise in order to achieve aerobic benefits is three sessions per week. For greater aerobic benefit, exercise five times per week.

6. Participating in a 50-minute to 60-minute aerobic dance class three to five times per week will help you meet most of your fitness goals.

7. To get the proper duration of exercise:
- You must do at least 5 continuous minutes of exercise at one time for each component of fitness.
- You must do a minimum of 20 continuous minutes of concentrated effort, in your target heart rate zone, for the cardiovascular component.

8. Factors known to increase the risks of cardiovascular disease are:
- a family history of heart disease
- high blood pressure
- cigarette smoking
- being overweight
- high levels of triglycerides and cholesterol in the blood
- diabetes
- stress
- physical inactivity

---

[4]Copyright © 1998 American Heart Association Inc. American Heart Association publications, 1998–2000.

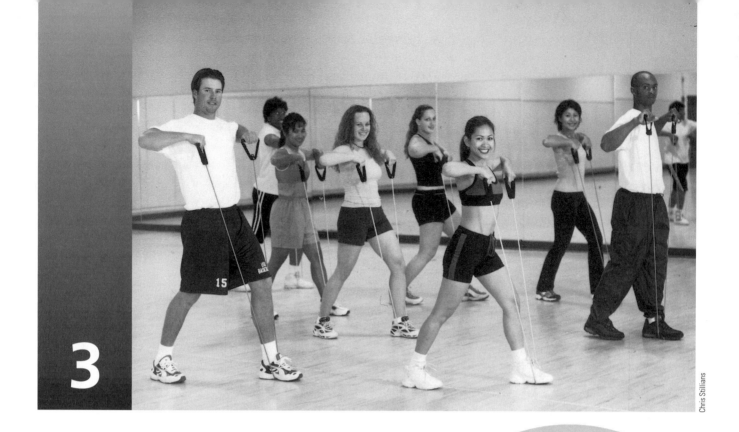

Chris Stillians

3

Committing Yourself to a Workout

Outline

Benefits of an Aerobic Exercise
Class
Components of a Good Class
Checklist for Your First Aerobics
Class
Warm-Up and Stretching
Checklist for Warm-Up
Cardiovascular/Aerobics Work

Strengthening and Toning Work
Cool-Down and Flexibility
Frequency of Workouts
How Long Before Results Are
Apparent?
What to Wear to Class
Selecting Shoes
Summary

To get the benefit from exercising, specifically from aerobics, you must stick with it! Exercising must become an integral part of your weekly routine. You need to be convinced of the benefits you will derive from it, and then you will make exercising a part of your lifestyle. Schedule your aerobics class into your life, and don't allow other things to interrupt this commitment.

Benefits of an Aerobic Exercise Class

There are physiological, psychological, and social benefits of an aerobic dance exercise class. The physiological benefits, as discussed in the last chapter, are numerous. The heart muscle strengthens and becomes more efficient as it pumps more blood. Lung capacity increases, and muscle fibers increase in size and perform more efficiently. The number of red blood cells increases. Bones become stronger, denser, and more resistant to deterioration. Weight control is aided because the metabolic rate is elevated for several hours after exercise, and more calories are burned during exercise. Also, digestion and elimination are improved.

A psychological benefit is a feeling of well-being after exercise. Research suggests that during exercise a euphoria-producing chemical called encephalin is released. Brain cells release similar substances called endorphins, which produce a feeling of well-being and relaxation. In addition, you feel better when you know you are doing something good for yourself. Once you start looking better and seeing results from exercise, you will feel better during and after class.

A social benefit is that you meet people in an aerobic dance class. Having familiar faces and people to talk to before and after a class helps keep you motivated to continue exercising. Also, you receive emotional support from your friends to continue your exercise program. You probably know the saying "misery loves company." If you miss an aerobics class, you can be sure

someone will ask you where you were. Another important social aspect is that exercising is more fun in groups. If you are having fun exercising, you are more likely to make the activity a regular part of your life.

Components of a Good Class

All good aerobics or dance exercise classes have four parts:

1. warm-up and stretching
2. cardiovascular/aerobics work
3. strengthening and toning work
4. cool-down and flexibility

It is important to participate in all four parts of the class as they are designed to prepare your body for the work you are doing in a progressive, safe manner. Also, to get the best results from working out, you need to work on all components of conditioning.

Many people associate a good workout with pain. You've undoubtedly heard the phrase "no pain, no gain." Popular media reinforces such an erroneous concept. You will experience some discomforts during and after a good class: some mild aches and soreness, perhaps a slight shortness of breath, and a feeling of fatigue. But these discomforts are minor and temporary. Be careful, because if you feel pain when you exercise, this is a sign of overexercising (or overexertion), and you will need to moderate your activity. A good aerobics class offers activities that will not hurt you. However, you must always protect yourself and understand and respect the signs your body gives you.

Warm-Up and Stretching

The warm-up portion of class usually lasts 7 to 10 minutes. The purpose is to activate your circulatory system and progressively prepare your body for the upcoming high-intensity activities. During warm-up, your heart rate gradually increases, circulation improves, ventilation increases, oxygen flow increases, muscles and joints warm-up and become more flexible, and stiffness and soreness are reduced. Additionally, a warm-up

Checklist for Your First Aerobics Class

1. Are you the type of person who sticks to something from the start, or do you drop out before the job is done? If you are the former, then you will easily commit yourself to a workout.

2. To benefit from exercise, you must stick with it.

3. Make a schedule of your weekly commitments. Find a window of time to fit regular exercise into your schedule.

4. The three facets of life where aerobic dance exercise will benefit you are in the physiological, psychological, and social parts of your life.

5. The four components of a good class are:
   - warm-up and stretching
   - aerobics/cardiovascular work
   - strengthening and toning work
   - cool-down and flexibility

6. Remember, "No pain, no gain" is an erroneous concept.

7. You should work out 3 to 5 times per week at such an adequate intensity as to achieve cardiovascular fitness.

8. Do not become discouraged: remember that it will take approximately 8 weeks to see the visible results of your hard work through exercise.

9. Wear comfortable clothes to class that allow your body to breathe. Do not wear nylon, rubber, or non-permeable clothes.

10. Select shoes that are meant for aerobic exercising. They should be comfortable, provide you with good support, and have impact-absorption qualities.

mentally prepares you to fully participate in the dance exercise class. Tension gradually subsides during that time because of the rhythmic movement.

The warm-up also includes stretching. It is very important that you perform static stretches (or stretches that are sustained for a period of time without extra movement) and that you hold your stretches for 10 to 30 seconds. Do not participate in bouncing, or what is called ballistic stretching. Ballistic stretching can lead to the tearing of muscles. Each person has a different degree of flexibility. Know your capabilities and be aware of your limitations. If you feel discomfort or extreme tightness, release the stretch you are in and do not stretch any further in that position. Another very important point to remember is that when you warm your body up progressively and properly, you reduce the potential for injury. It is imperative that you arrive on time to your aerobics class so that you don't miss the warm-up.

Cardiovascular/ Aerobics Work

The aerobic portion of the class begins slowly, and progressively increases in intensity to gradually overload your circulatory system. The length varies from 12 to 30 minutes depending on the overall length and level of the class. The aerobic routines incorporate a variety of movements designed to use all parts of the body and to raise the heart rate to its target zone. Between movement phases, or every 5 to 10 minutes, monitor your pulse to determine if you are working at the correct intensity to maintain your target heart rate.

The purpose of the cardiovascular/ aerobic phase of class is to:

1. elevate the heart rate to the target zone, and keep it there for 12 to 30 minutes

2. strengthen the heart muscle

3. stress the circulatory system, which yields cardiovascular endurance

4. improve and increase muscular endurance

5. improve and increase lung ventilation

A post-aerobic cool-down is extremely important. It is wise to end the aerobic section of class with approximately 2 to 3 minutes of slower-paced movements. During this period, the heart rate and blood pressure return to a more stable level before you proceed to floor work. At the end of this brief cool-down period,

Checklist for Warm-Up

Begin your warm-up activities with a progressively paced, gentle form of aerobic activity to "start your circulation moving," so to speak. For example, you could begin by slowly walking around the room and gradually walking faster until you reach a jogging pace. You could also increase your heart rate by performing jumping jacks or running in place slowly to music. Continue this type of overall body warm-up for approximately 2 to 3 minutes. Then begin stretching activities. A well-designed aerobics class incorporates this type of warm-up into the early part of the class.

Stretching

Stretch each large muscle group in your body slowly. Hold each stretch for approximately 20 seconds.

1. Legs
   - _____ Hamstrings (back of the thighs)
   - _____ Quadriceps (front of the thighs)
   - _____ Abductors (outside of the thighs and hips)
   - _____ Adductors (inside of the thighs and hips)
   - _____ Gastrocnemius (calf muscle)
   - _____ Tibialis anterior (muscle in front of leg, below the knee)
2. Back
   - _____ Upper back
   - _____ Lower back
3. Abdominals
   - _____ Front
   - _____ Sides
4. Shoulders
5. Neck

---

your heart rate should be at or under 60 percent of your maximum heart rate.

Strengthening and Toning Work

A good instructor makes a smooth transition to the floor to begin strengthening and conditioning. The purpose of this phase, which lasts approximately 10 to 20 minutes, is to increase the strength, endurance, tone, and flexibility of your muscles. A good instructor leads exercises that work the entire body. A concentrated effort is made to increase the muscular strength and endurance of the biceps, triceps, thighs, abdomen, abdominal muscles, and buttocks (gluteals).

Upon approaching the floor, you may find yourself a little light-headed. If so, tell your instructor. You may need to walk around the room a while in order to lower your heart rate more gradually.

Cool-Down and Flexibility

The purpose of the cool-down and flexibility phase is to allow the body to gradually recover from the stress placed on it during your high-intensity workout. Cooling down serves two purposes:

1. To ease you out of your aerobic and strengthening activity at a slow pace in order to allow your heart rate to return to normal.

2. To stretch your muscles so that injury and stiffening are prevented. If you stop exercising suddenly, you may cause a pooling of blood in the lower legs. This may result in dizziness or a light-headed feeling.

At the end of class, you should perform slow, steady stretching for a minimum of 5 minutes to redistribute the blood flow equally and return the body to its pre-exercise state. After 5 to 10 minutes of cool-down, your heart rate should be close to 100 beats per minute. Remember that warm muscles stretch best. Perform static stretches and hold all of your stretches for approximately 10 to 30 seconds.

Frequency of Workouts

Research indicates that working out with adequate intensity three to five times per week is all that is necessary to achieve cardiovascular fitness. You don't have to knock yourself out 7 days per week. It is important physiologically and psychologically to allow yourself a 24- to 48-hour recovery each week. Attending an aerobics class three to five times per week will keep you in good shape.

How Long Before Results Are Apparent?

Improved fitness and changes in your appearance take time, so don't become discouraged if you don't see a change in your body after only one week of working out. Research indicates that people participating in a vigorous physical exercise program experience increased efficiency in their cardiovascular system in approximately 8 weeks. However, after a few weeks, you will notice an improvement in your lung capacity. This will yield less breathlessness during the aerobic section of class. You may also begin to feel a little more flexible and stronger. Allow your body time to change, adjust, and improve. Before long you will see changes in your body that will reinforce your efforts.

What to Wear to Class

Comfortable clothes that provide ease of movement along with a good pair of aerobic or athletic shoes are all that you need. Generally, students wear leotards and tights, T-shirts and shorts, or warm-up suits. Cotton or a cotton-mix fabric provides the most comfort. Cotton "breathes" and helps your body maintain its normal temperature by pulling perspiration away from the skin. With warm-up suits, you perspire so much that you become too hot. If you do wear a warm-up suit, wear clothes underneath it so you can remove the top and/or bottom of the suit when you get too warm. Nylon, rubber, or nonpermeable clothes are not recommended because they trap heat and prevent the evaporation of perspiration.

Selecting Shoes

A good aerobics shoe not only feels good, but it also may help prevent injury. It is important to buy shoes that are lightweight and supportive, can move with your foot, and can absorb shock. Shoes that do not absorb impact make you more susceptible to Achilles' tendonitis, shin splints, knee pain, foot pain, and stress fractures.

The right midsole of the shoe can offset the stresses that may lead to injury. The most popular material used in the midsoles, ethylene vinyl acetate (EVA), offers the best structure for absorbing shock. The ability of the shoe's midsole to dampen the force of impact is measured in durometers. The higher the rating, the firmer the sole and the greater its shock-absorbing ability. The taller and heavier you are, the firmer the midsole you need. Shoes also come with cushioning cartridges to absorb impact and better support your foot. When first selecting aerobics shoes, seek the advice of a knowledgeable shoe salesperson. Shoe manufacturers change designs frequently to meet market demands. A salesperson can best advise you on the advantages of one brand of aerobics shoe over another.

You need to decide whether to buy high-top, mid-cut, or low-cut shoes. The difference is individual. However, some people have weak ankles and choose the high- or mid-top shoe because it provides more ankle support. Other people prefer a low-cut aerobics shoe.

Some people put pads or orthotics inside their shoes to add support and/or cushioning. Ask your shoe salesperson about pads or try them out yourself.

It is important to buy a shoe made for aerobic exercising if this is your main fitness activity. Some shoes are called "cross trainer" shoes. These are designed for exercisers who regularly participate in running, weight training, Kick Boxing, etc. as well as aerobics. Determine your needs, discuss them with a salesperson, and try out the shoe for as long as you can in the store. It is a mistake to just put on a shoe and buy it. Once the shoe is on, stand up, walk around, perform some of the movements you do in class, and decide whether you like the shoe. Trying on the shoe and seeing how it fits and supports you is the most important step in selecting the correct exercise shoe.

Once you have found the most comfortable and supportive shoe appropriate for your fitness routine, you should buy the shoe. This shoe may last you 3 to 6 months, depending on the frequency in which you wear it for exercising. If the shoe "breaks down" and loses the cushioning and supporting qualities for which you bought it, then you could be prone to injury. Indicators of a shoe that needs to be replaced include stretching of the shoe, rolled-over heels, a loosening of the shoe, and pain in your feet. You need to pay attention to the condition of your shoes and replace them as needed.

Summary

1. There are physiological, psychological, and social benefits from an aerobic dance exercise class.

2. To gain the benefits of an aerobics class, you must make exercise an integral part of your weekly routine.

3. Aerobic exercise provides the following physiological benefits:
   - The number of red blood cells increases.
   - The heart muscle strengthens and becomes more efficient as it pumps more blood with each stroke.
   - Lung capacity increases.
   - Bones become stronger and more dense.
   - The metabolic rate is elevated for several hours after exercise, thereby aiding in weight control.
   - Digestion and elimination are improved.

4. Psychological benefits also are a reward of aerobic dance exercise.

5. Following an aerobics class, people usually have a sense of well-being.

6. The components of a good class are warm-up, aerobics, strengthening and toning, cool-down, and flexibility.

7. Working out with adequate intensity three to five times per week yields cardiovascular fitness.

8. Improved fitness and changes in your physical appearance take time. Research indicates that it takes approximately eight weeks to experience increased efficiency in your cardiovascular system.

9. Remember, it is important physiologically and psychologically to allow yourself a 24- to 48-hour recovery each week.

10. Many people make the mistake of leaving class before they have completed a cool-down. Remember the two phases to a cool-down are:
    - to slowly return your heart rate to normal.
    - to stretch your muscles to prevent injury and stiffening.

11. Go to class physically, emotionally, and practically prepared to work out.

12. Wear permeable, comfortable clothes and supportive shoes. You don't need to be a fashion plate to participate in an aerobic dance exercise class!

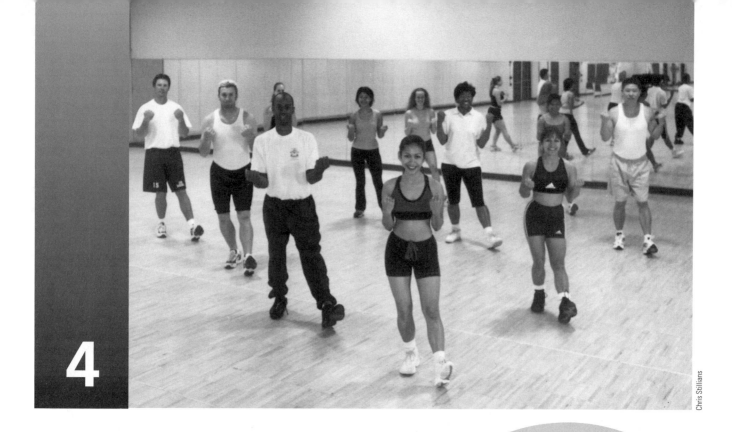

Chris Stillians

Motivation

Outline

Negative Motivation
Positive Motivation
Inner-Directed versus Outer-
    Directed
Why You Keep Going
Checklist for Mental Benefits
    of Aerobics
Setting Personal Goals

Following the Goals with Action
Checklist for Personal Goal
    Setting
Visualization
Checklist for Mental Imagery
Additional Tips to Keep You
    Motivated
Summary

The desire to become physically fit through aerobic exercise is often evident when people begin a regular exercise program; however, the desire may not be strong enough to sustain them through a long-term commitment. In order to stick with a program, exercisers can benefit from a variety of motivating tips and techniques.

Motivation refers to an inner drive that compels you to behave a certain way. You can be motivated to either pursue or avoid something. *Aversion therapy* is an example of training the mind and body to be repelled by a negative addiction, such as smoking or alcohol. *Incentive therapy* refers to the rewarding of something pleasurable after the accomplishment of a certain positive behavior; for instance, receiving the keys to the family car for improving your grades.

This chapter contains some current thinking about motivation from the realm of the sport psychologist. It can be used to help you think about your own motivation as an aerobic exerciser.

Negative Motivation

The motivational technique that may have worked at one time for you will not necessarily motivate you several months down the road. Your attitudes and beliefs about what motivates you are in a constant state of change and adjustment. As you achieve certain short- and long-term goals, the elements of what spurred you on in the beginning no longer hold true at a later date.

The simplest way to identify your source of motivation is to identify and understand your particular needs. Here is an example: Steve is a 24-year-old computer programmer with a sedentary lifestyle and no great love of sports. He is gaining weight steadily and finds himself about 25 pounds overweight. He is surprised to discover that he can't climb the stairs to his apartment without being short of breath. The slightest activity seems to wear him out. As he takes a physical inventory, he realizes he is fast becoming as out of shape as his father,

who died at the age of 43 from a heart attack. The fear of dying at such a young age scares Steve into signing up at a local health club. He dives feet first into a 6-day-a-week jogging program, develops shin splints from doing too much too fast, and starts to grow discouraged that the weight isn't coming off as fast as he'd like.

The push behind Steve's desire to exercise arose from a negative source: fear of heart disease and death. Negative motivation isn't without its usefulness. It did get Steve started in the right direction. Many of us experience negative motivation in our everyday lives. For example, you may go on a diet because you "can't stand this body anymore." An eight-year-old finally stops sucking her thumb because she is not going to let "those brats call me a baby anymore."

The negative motivation that drove Steve into exercising also drove him into an overuse syndrome, where he did not approach his fitness regimen with a realistic plan. A painful case of shin splints could keep Steve from exercising for several weeks, long enough to set up a cycle of despair, feelings of failure, complete inactivity, and more weight gain. Overcoming the obstacles to exercise may be more difficult the second time around for Steve.

The problem with negative motivation is that although it may be useful in the beginning, it is often not enough of an impetus to keep you going for a lifetime commitment. Negative motivation makes you run *from* something, but not necessarily *to* anything. If the negative event or feeling that originally triggered the action starts to fade as a memory or grow distant in time, there will not be enough fuel to keep the wheels in motion.

Positive Motivation

Positive motivation refers to attitudes, beliefs, and traits that spring from a source that enhances your performance, outlook, and confidence about exercise. Although it is more difficult to experience positive motivation in the initial stages of aerobic exercise, the nature of positive motivation is more sustaining in the long run. Here is an example:

Paula is a 20-year-old college senior who has devoted all her energy to

Assessing your condition for motivation

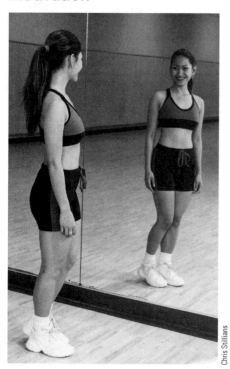

Chris Stillians

studying and passing her final examinations. She admits to letting her body "fall apart," to surviving on junk food, very little sleep, and a complete lack of exercise. Now that she has to enter the career market, she wants to clean up her act, as she says, and get in shape for job interviews. As she starts taking aerobics classes three times a week, she finds they are tougher than she thought they would be. However, she is determined to achieve her goals of a 5-pound weight loss in 1 month, a firmer physique in 3 months, and more energy.

Paula keeps a weekly log of the time, intensity, and frequency of her participation in aerobics classes, and also records her weight and activities each week. After 3 weeks, she is surprised to find that her eating patterns are starting to change. The desire to load up on high-fat, fast foods is starting to diminish. It's beginning to seem pointless to her to work so hard in exercise class, and then counteract all her good efforts with one quick fix of a greasy burger, fries, and milkshake. The aerobics class is becoming a little easier, but she remembers how tough it was in the beginning.

Paula is not alone. Sports psychologists have studied a transference of positive health habits to other lifestyle aspects among first-time exercisers. People who become committed to their exercise programs tend to cut down on smoking, eat a more nutritious diet, and reduce alcohol and substance abuse.

Positive motivation is self-reinforcing behavior that allows you to continue an action because of the rewarding benefits that slowly become evident. The human body was not made to be inactive, but rather, to be physically used. When we exercise regularly, the bones, muscles, heart, lungs, and blood vessels all begin to function better. If we do not stimulate our bodies into physical action, all of its functional capacities begin to decline at an accelerated rate. We begin to grow old before our time. When the benefits of regular exercise, both psychological and physical, begin to kick in (anywhere from 3 to 12 weeks after starting a program) positive motivation can take over the incentive job from the ini-

tial negative motivation. Positive or intrinsic motivation can last a lifetime.

Inner-Directed versus Outer-Directed

Have you ever known a person who is self-motivated? Self-motivated people are often the subjects of studies on exercise adherence. The personality traits that distinguish someone who is self-motivated are categorized and logged by researchers. One such trait is his or her ability to easily dismiss the types of excuses used by other individuals to not exercise: they don't look good that day, the class is too crowded, or they don't feel like going alone. Self-motivated people are inner-directed; their goals come from an inner source instead of from others, such as family and friends.

Outer-directed individuals exercise because their boyfriend or girlfriend wants them to get in shape, because their friends joined a club, or because they want to please someone else. The chances of staying with an exercise program are lower for the outer-directed than for the inner-directed person. Because there is no conscious awareness attached to the exercise, the outer-directed person does not always look forward to the benefits, and often drops out of the program before any real gains are made. It is possible for the outer-directed individual to shift to being an inner-directed exerciser. Think of someone you know who started exercising to attract someone's attention, but continued with the program regardless of whether the original motivator was still on the scene.

Why You Keep Going

What really keeps you going in an exercise program? What makes you lace up your aerobic shoes for one more class,

Checklist for Mental Benefits of Aerobics

Research in the last two decades has led investigators to conclude that there are mental benefits associated with aerobics. These include:

1. overall improvement in self-esteem
2. improved ability to cope with stress and tension
3. less free-floating anxiety
4. enhanced ability to concentrate and focus on one issue at a time
5. increased confidence about reaching goals
6. greater sense of self-acceptance
7. greater sense of satisfaction
8. overall improvement in mood
9. increased ability to relax

even on days when you're dragging your heels? Research shows that for many people, the physical benefit of exercise is stimulus enough to keep them going. For others, the psychological benefits weigh more heavily. But for the majority, a sense of well-being and a positive glow following exercise tends to keep them positively addicted to their aerobic regimens.

Traditionally, exercise scientists have looked to the "runner's high" as a reason for long-term adherence. The "runner's high," reported by millions of aerobics enthusiasts, is a feeling of elation and uplifted spirits that lasts 2 to 6 hours after a vigorous exercise session.

Physiologically, it follows from the release of a neurochemical transmitter, known as endorphin, which affects the body in a way similar to morphine. All sensation of pain or discomfort is masked, and a feeling of expansive self-worth occurs.

Today, some scientists are reporting that a psychological addiction to exercise kicks in, with or without the release of endorphins, and that the positive mental attachment to the entire lifestyle of fitness is what keeps people coming back for more. In any case, the mental benefits of aerobics carry their own motivational message.

Many of these mental benefits can enhance your physical performance during aerobics. The improvement in focus and concentration is a good example. By increasing the amount of resistance that you apply to contracting muscles during the floor work session of an aerobics class, you can actually increase the workload of that area, thereby increas-

ing strength, muscular endurance, and total caloric burn. Another example of a mental benefit having an impact on performance is the ability to relax. Rest is an important part of physical training and can lay the groundwork for progression to the next level of goal achievement.

Setting Personal Goals

The setting of goals and working toward their accomplishment is a significant part of all exercise programs, and aerobics is no exception. Goal setting also goes hand-in-hand with motivational techniques. The gratifying sense of achievement that follows when a goal is accomplished scores high marks as a motivational tool. The success can be transferred into all other areas of life that impact your exercise regimen, reinforcing the next wave of goals and efforts.

Goals for an aerobics program might include:

1. to gain both strength and cardiovascular endurance

2. to develop more power

3. to gain greater flexibility

4. to lose excess fat

5. to lower the resting heart rate

6. to sleep more soundly due to the right amount of physical fatigue

7. to perfect a new choreography

Following the Goals with Action

Motivation centers on the intensity and extent of your desire to accomplish a

Checklist for Personal Goal Setting

In the chart below, list the personal goals you would like to attain upon completion of this class:

List Your Personal Goals Below	Date You Would Like To Accomplish These Goals
1.	
2.	
3.	
4.	
5.	

goal. The amount of enthusiasm you have in pursuing a goal indicates how much you really want to achieve that goal. Many people say they want to accomplish a goal, but only by looking at how fervently they pursue it can we accurately measure their desire for a positive outcome. In other words, talk is cheap. It's not enough to say "I want to get in shape." With aerobic exercise, the action versus the expression is what counts; it's what you do, not what you say.

Visualization

The practice of imagery or mental visualization is a technique that has been useful in motivating athletes to improve performance. The technique was pioneered by the European sports coaches and has been successfully employed by sports professionals and enthusiasts everywhere.

During mental visualization, the participant closes his or her eyes (usually) and envisions the actual performance of a sport or activity, with perfect execution, and a successful win or out-

come. Greg Louganis, a former U.S. Olympic champion diver, used visualization to rehearse dives, as did many other successful professional and amateur athletes.

As an aerobic exerciser, you can mentally practice your routine by seeing yourself performing the moves correctly. An advanced imagery technique allows you to move the action internally so that instead of closing your eyes and watching yourself do something, you try to imagine others watching you flawlessly execute a perfect high-energy routine of a 60-minute class.

The technique of visualization works as a motivational technique because it helps you embrace the concept of yourself as a competent aerobic exerciser. Once you think of yourself as successful at something, you begin to adopt new attitudes and beliefs about yourself. This is part of the new "you." You can do this easily and with total enjoyment and have the ability to derive lifelong benefits from aerobics. Your motivation increases in proportion to your successful achievement of the task or routine.

✔ *Checklist for Mental Imagery*

1. See yourself from the outside as you practice a movement. Is your technique correct?

2. Feel your imaginary movement from the inside. Imagine yourself lasting the full 35 minutes of the aerobics workout even when you're tired.

3. Close your eyes and self-evaluate yourself. Do you feel you perform and

exercise with inner-directed motivation or outer-directed motivation?

4. If you identified your motivation to be outer-directed motivation, what is it specifically that motivates you to exercise regularly? When you focus on that motivator, do you perform better? If so, imagine that source of motivation before you begin your exercise routine.

Additional Tips to Keep You Motivated

Researchers have found that people who exercise at the same time every day are more likely to stick with an exercise program than people who vary their time. Another successful motivational technique is to find an exercise buddy. If the social context of exercise is friendly and inviting, the positive feelings are reinforcing. Finally, using a progress log and recognizing your achievement are highly motivational.

Summary

1. Try to identify a particular need for exercise. Look for something that can be solved or improved through regular exercise.

2. Beginning exercisers can be driven to launch a program because of negative motivation. Although useful, this is often not enough to lead them to a long-term commitment.

3. Positive motivation arises from the self-reinforcing benefits of exercise, both physical and psychological.

4. The inner-directed exerciser is someone who is self-motivated and overcomes common barriers to working out.

5. Outer-directed individuals may exercise because of someone else (or something else) in the early days, but can switch their source of motivation to inner-directed attitudes.

6. The psychological benefits of exercise coupled with the release of endorphins create a strong motivational force.

7. Setting and achieving goals for exercise can trigger feelings of success and self-worth throughout your life.

8. Visualization is a method of mentally rehearsing an ideal performance.

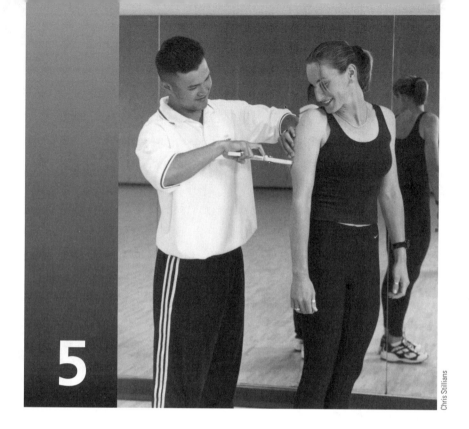

Chris Stillians

Assessing Your Fitness Level

Outline

What Condition Are You In Now?

Assessing Your Personal
    Measurements

Testing Your Aerobic Capacity
  3-Minute Step Test (Aerobic
    Assessment)

Testing Your General Flexibility

Student Health History

Summary

Checklist: Semester Progress
    Chart

What Condition Are You In Now?

What condition are you in now? You may look pretty good in the mirror, but are you aerobically fit? Perhaps you are, but you may be carrying a few extra pounds that you would like to shed. It is important to evaluate your current fitness level so that you: (1) are aware of your current status, and (2) can measure your progress. There is nothing better than seeing progress to help you stick with and enjoy a regular exercise program.

When you begin an exercise program, the initial discomforts of fatigue, soreness, dry mouth, and labored breathing seem discouraging. Try to remember there is no such thing as instant fitness. The benefits take about 6 to 12 weeks to appear. You must commit yourself to your exercise program. Unfortunately, if you are not committed and persistent, you may drop out before the results are apparent. There is an easy

way to visualize your progress. Gains, even small ones, can be measured right from the start. When you begin a new exercise program, take a good look at yourself in the mirror and assess your current fitness level so you can easily assess your progress. Becoming aware of your progress is a self-motivator and will help you stick to your exercise program. The three areas in which you can easily perform a self-assessment are personal measurements, aerobic conditioning, and flexibility.

Assessing Your Personal Measurements

It is sometimes difficult to take your own measurements due to the awkward angles. Try to find a trusted friend to help you out and complete the following chart. If not, take your own measurements. Complete the chart: (1) before you begin your new aerobic exercise program, (2) after 4 weeks into your exercise program, (3) after 8 weeks, (4) after 12 weeks, and (5) after 16 weeks. You will be amazed at your progress!

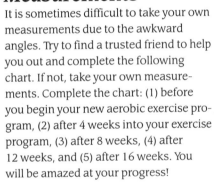

Assessing Your Personal Measurements*

Area of Measurement	Beginning Date Right	Left	4 weeks Date Right	Left	8 weeks Date Right	Left	12 weeks Date Right	Left	16 weeks Date Right	Left
Biceps/Triceps (upper arm midway between the elbow and shoulder joint)										
Chest										
Waist										
Hips (7″ below the waist)										
Upper Thigh (feet approx. 12″ apart; measure thighs 3″ below crotch level)										
Calf										

*Note: Record your measurement to the closest 1/2 inch.

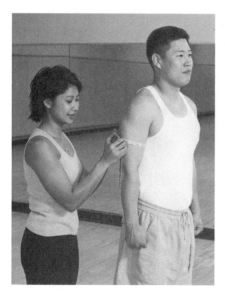

a. Measuring the biceps/triceps area

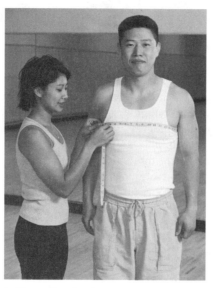

b. Measuring the chest

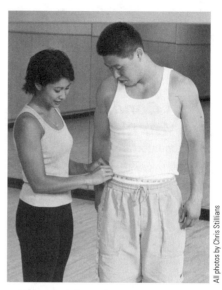

c. Measuring the waist

Testing Your Aerobic Capacity

It is a good idea to test your aerobic capacity using the 3-Minute Step Test when beginning your aerobic conditioning class or program. The 3-Minute Step Test that you can perform at home with a friend or at the facility where you are taking your aerobics class is listed below.

3-Minute Step Test (Aerobic Assessment)—

The purpose of the Step Test is to measure your heart rate in the recovery period following 3 minutes of stepping. If you cannot finish the test, or score at the very poor level, you should obtain medical clearance before further testing. This should not be performed if you are taking a beta blocker medication (or any other medication affecting heart rate).

Training Heart Rates Chart					
Heart Beats per Minute				**Your score:** _____	
Age	**Very High**	**High**	**Moderate**	**Low**	**Very Low**
Female					
10–19	Below 82	82–91	92–97	98–102	Above 102
20–29	Below 83	83–87	88–93	94–98	Above 98
30–39	Below 83	82–89	90–95	96–98	Above 98
40–49	Below 83	82–87	88–97	98–102	Above 102
Over 50	Below 86	86–93	94–99	100–104	Above 104
Male					
10–19	Below 72	72–77	78–83	84–88	Above 89
20–29	Below 72	72–79	80–85	86–93	Above 94
30–39	Below 76	76–81	82–87	88–93	Above 94
40–49	Below 78	78–83	84–89	90–94	Above 95
Over 50	Below 80	80–85	86–91	92–95	Above 96

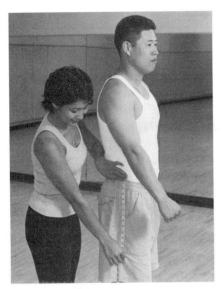

a. Locating 7″ below waist for hip measurement

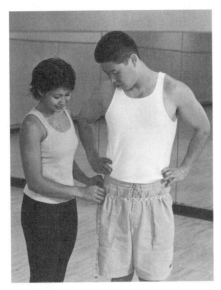

b. Hip measurement

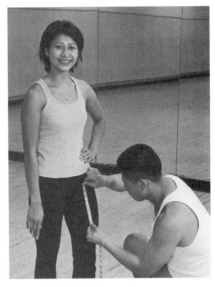

c. Locating 3″ below crotch for thigh measurement

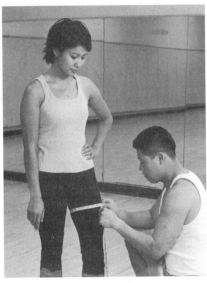

d. Upper thigh measurement

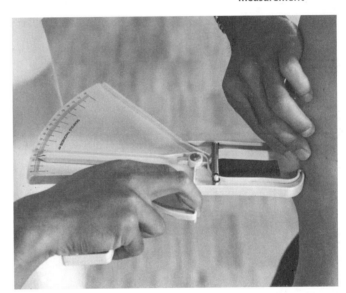

e. Skin calipers testing of tricep area

Equipment Needed:

- a 12-inch step

- stop watch (or watch displaying seconds) for timing the test and counting recovery heart rate

- metronome to set cadence (may use pre-recorded audio cassette tape and player)

Procedure:

- You should warm-up before beginning this test.

- Step up and down at a rate of 24 steps per minute (metronome setting of 96) for 3 minutes.

- Immediately after the 3 minutes of stepping, sit down on a chair or bench and find your pulse (at the neck). Take a 60-second heart rate 5 seconds after the completion of stepping.

- This recovery heart rate is the score. Consult the standards in the chart below to determine your fitness category.

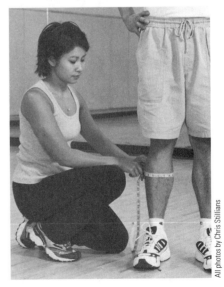

f. Measuring the calf

All photos by Chris Stillians

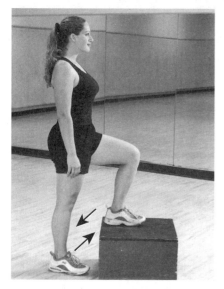

a. Step test

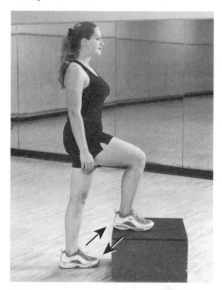

b. Step test

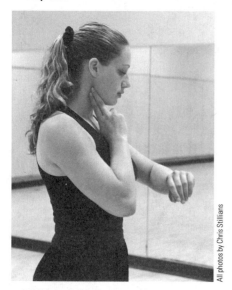

c. Taking pulse following step test

All photos by Chris Stillians

US Army Center for Health Promotion and Preventive Medicine

3-Minute Aerobic Step Test
(Men & Women)

Category	Gender	Heart Rate
Excellent	male	< 71
	female	< 97
Good	male	71–102
	female	97–127
Fair	male	103–117
	female	128–142
Poor	male	118–147
	female	143–171
Very Poor	male	148+
	female	172+

From Kasch, F.W. and J.L. Boyer. *Adult Fitness Principles and Practices.* San Diego State College, San Diego, 1968.

Interpreting your Results:

If your score is within the good-to-excellent categories, congratulations and keep up the good work! If you are in the fair rating category, there is room for improvement in your cardiovascular respiratory endurance level. If your score falls within the very poor or poor rating, a regular aerobic program will make a big difference in your cardiovascular respiratory endurance level.

Testing Your General Flexibility

Flexibility is specific to a certain joint or a combination of joints. With extensive testing, you can have the flexibility in every joint evaluated and identified. However, you can measure your general flexibility by using the Sit-and-Reach Test. To perform this test, you need a Sit-and-Reach Box. Ask your instructor where you can find one, or you can build one yourself.

Directions:

Sit with the soles of your feet flat against the Sit-and-Reach Box. Keeping your knees straight, reach forward with your arms fully extended, palms down, fingers straight, and one hand on top of the other. Hold this position for 3 seconds, determining the longest length of your reach. Repeat and use the best score.

Compare your score to the following chart to assess your flexibility.

Flexibility (Women) Sit-and-Reach: Inches

				Age			
%	< 20	20–29	30–39	40–49	50–59	60+	
99	> 24.3	> 24.0	> 24.0	> 22.8	> 23.0	> 23.0	
95	24.3	24.0	24.0	22.8	23.0	23.0	S
90	24.3	23.8	22.5	21.5	21.5	21.8	
85	22.5	23.0	22.0	21.3	21.0	19.5	
80	22.5	22.5	21.5	20.5	20.3	19.0	E
75	22.3	22.0	21.0	20.0	20.0	18.0	
70	22.0	21.5	20.5	19.8	19.3	17.5	
65	21.8	21.0	20.3	19.1	19.0	17.5	
60	21.5	20.5	20.0	19.0	18.5	17.0	G
55	21.3	20.3	19.5	18.5	18.0	17.0	
50	21.0	20.0	19.0	18.0	17.9	16.4	
45	20.5	19.5	18.5	18.0	17.0	16.1	
40	20.5	19.3	18.3	17.3	16.8	15.5	F
35	20.0	19.0	17.8	17.0	16.0	15.2	
30	19.5	18.3	17.3	16.5	15.5	14.4	
25	19.0	17.8	16.8	16.0	15.3	13.6	
20	18.5	17.0	16.5	15.0	14.8	13.0	P
15	17.8	16.4	15.5	14.0	14.0	11.5	
10	14.5	15.4	14.4	13.0	13.0	11.5	
5	14.5	14.1	12.0	10.5	12.3	9.2	VP
1	< 14.5	< 14.1	< 12.0	< 10.5	< 12.3	< 9.2	

S = superior	E = excellent	G = good	F = fair	P = poor	VP = very poor

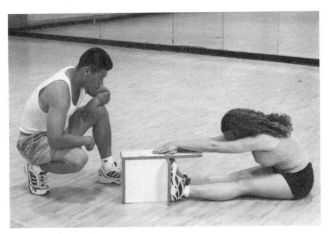

a. Reading score of sit and reach test

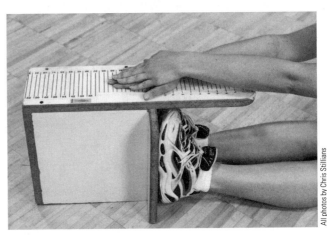

b. Sit and reach test

All photos by Chris Stillians

Flexibility (Men) Sit-and-Reach: Inches

%	< 20	20–29	30–39	40–49	50–59	60 +	
			Age				
99	> 23.4	> 23.0	> 22.0	> 21.3	> 20.5	> 20.0	
95	23.4	23.0	22.0	21.3	20.5	20.0	S
90	22.6	21.8	21.0	20.0	19.0	19.0	
85	22.4	21.0	20.0	19.3	18.3	18.0	
80	21.7	20.5	19.5	18.5	17.5	17.3	E
75	21.4	20.0	19.0	18.0	17.0	16.5	
70	20.7	19.5	18.5	17.5	16.5	15.5	
65	19.8	19.0	18.0	17.0	16.0	15.0	
60	19.0	18.5	17.5	16.3	15.5	14.5	G
55	18.7	18.0	17.0	16.0	15.0	14.0	
50	18.0	17.5	16.5	15.3	14.5	13.5	
45	17.3	17.0	16.0	15.0	14.0	13.0	
40	16.5	16.5	15.5	14.3	13.3	12.5	F
35	16.0	16.0	15.0	14.0	12.5	12.0	
30	15.5	15.5	14.5	13.3	12.0	11.3	
25	14.1	15.0	13.8	12.5	11.2	10.5	
20	13.2	14.4	13.0	12.0	10.5	10.0	P
15	11.9	13.5	12.0	11.0	9.7	9.0	
10	10.5	12.3	11.0	10.0	8.5	8.0	
5	9.4	10.5	9.3	8.3	7.0	5.8	VP
1	< 9.4	< 10.5	< 9.3	< 8.3	< 7.0	< 5.8	

S = superior   E = excellent   G = good   F = fair   P = poor   VP = very poor

Student Health History

Before you begin your aerobics program, it is important for your instructor to know something about your history to assist you if necessary. Please fill out the form below, and give it to your instructor by the second week of class.

Student Health History

Name _____   Age _____

Date _____   Class Section _____

1. Do you have any of the following illnesses/conditions?
   _____ Asthma   _____ Epilepsy   _____ Hypertension
   _____ Emphysema   _____ Diabetes   _____ Heart Disease
   _____ Chest pain or discomfort   _____ Pregnancy

2. Have you had any of the following within the past 2 years?
   _____ Heart attack   _____ Stroke
   _____ Heart surgery   _____ Back injury
   _____ General major surgery. If so, please specify _____

3. Do you smoke? _____ Yes   _____ No

4. Are you currently taking any medications? _____ Yes   _____ No
   If yes, please specify. _____

5. Are you currently under a doctor's care? _____ Yes   _____ No
   If yes, please specify the reason. _____

6. Date of your last physical examination. _____

7. Were any health problems discovered as the result of this exam?
   _____ Yes   _____ No
   If so, please describe. _____

8. According to your physician and/or charts, are you
   _____ Overweight   If so, by how much? _____
   _____ Underweight   If so, by how much? _____
   _____ Normal

9. Do you have any handicaps or current, chronic injuries that limit your physical
   abilities? _____ Yes   _____ No
   If so, please describe. _____

10. Please supply any additional information that might be helpful to your
    instructor. _____

11. What are your main goals of this class? (Rank them by placing a 1, 2, or 3 on
    the line next to your goal.)
    _____ Lose weight   _____ Stay the same   _____ Gain weight
    _____ Tone muscles   _____ Build muscles   _____ Lose inches
    _____ Increase cardiovascular fitness
    _____ Other (please describe)_____

Summary

1. You must assess your current fitness level in order to set goals for yourself and measure your progress.

2. Remember, there is no such thing as instant fitness. It takes 6 to 12 weeks of consistent participation in an aerobics class before you will see results.

3. Regularly fill out the chart entitled "Assessing Your Personal Measurements" so you can visualize your results.

4. Complete the 3-Minute Step Test several times throughout the semester to evaluate your aerobic fitness level. Watch your improvement!

5. Be sure to perform the Sit-and-Reach Test to see your progress.

6. Fill out the Semester Progress Chart at the appropriate time to get an overall view of your progress.

7. Now you are on the road to improving your fitness and feeling better. Congratulations!

✔ Checklist: Semester Progress Chart

It is valuable to identify your progress throughout the semester. Complete the following for each week listed.

Progress Chart

	Week 1		Week 8		Week 10		Week 15	
Weight								
Waist Measurement								
Upper Arm Measurement (Around bicep/tricep muscle area)	R	L	R	L	R	L	R	L
Thigh Measurement (3″ below crotch)								
Hip Measurement (7″ below waist)								
Resting Heart Rate								
Sit and Reach Flexibility								
Modified Step Test								
Maximum Number of Push-ups								
Number of Curl-ups in 1 Minute								

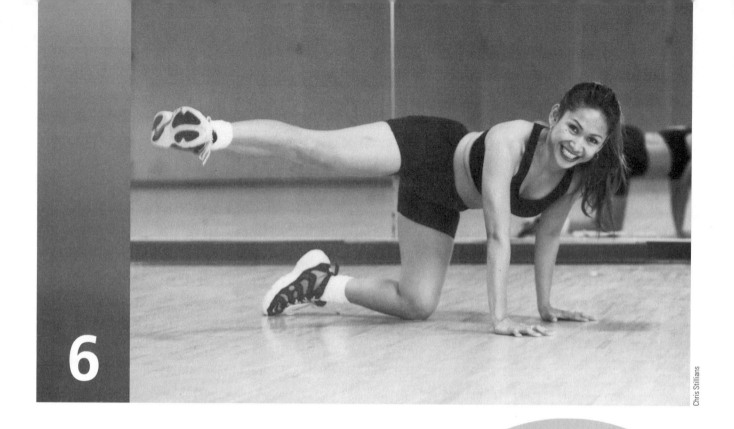

Chris Stillians

6

Your Personal Workout

Outline

Your Pre-Class Warm-Up

Stretches and Isolations
  Head Isolations
  Shoulder Circles
  Rib Isolations
  Rib Circles
  Hip Isolations
  Hip Circles
  Deep Lunge
  Side Lunge
  Hamstring Stretch
  Quadricep Stretch
  Calf Stretches
  Ankle Circles
  Ankle Raises

  Heel Walking
  Sitting Straddle Side Stretch
  Sitting Straddle Forward Stretch

Strengthening Exercises
  Push-Ups
  Reverse Push-Ups
  Abdominal Curl-Ups
  Donkey Leg Lifts
  Straight Leg Lifts
  Side Leg Lifts
  Bent Side Leg Lifts

Pelvic Lifts/Buttocks Exercise

Summary

Checklist for Your Personal
      Workout

Head isolations

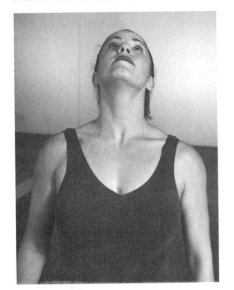

a. Up

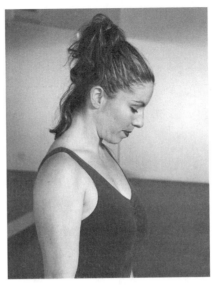

b. Down

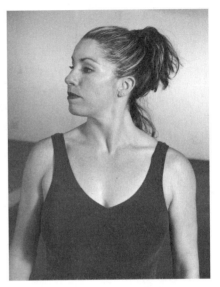

c. Side

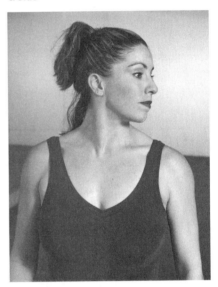

d. Side

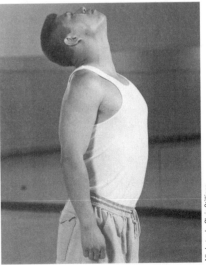

Caution: Hyperextension of neck can lead to injuries.

Once you have committed yourself to working out regularly, you must decide what you want to do for your weekly workout. Do you want to take an aerobics class four or five times per week? Or would you rather take a dance exercise class three times per week, while also walking and doing strengthening and flexibility exercises at home twice a week? Whatever you decide, you must stick to it to gain the benefits of exercising.

As mentioned in Chapter 1, aerobic exercise is defined as exercise that utilizes oxygen for a sustained activity of 2 minutes or longer. Even though aerobic dance exercise classes and jogging are what come to mind when you think of aerobics, there are other forms of viable aerobic exercise. They include brisk walking, race walking, swimming, rapid bicycling, rebounder ("mini" trampoline) exercising, jumping rope, aqua aerobics, cross-country skiing, and rowing-machine work. All these activities are usually done alone, with the exception of walking and bicycling. Many people drop out of solo-type activities in order to enjoy the group aspect of an aerobic dance exercise class. Remember, you must enjoy the type of activity you select to be able to stick to it. Decide how you like to exercise, in a group or alone, and create a weekly routine for yourself. Exercising regularly must be as habitual as brushing your teeth. Your mind and body will become accustomed to exercising at a certain time on particu-lar days and will miss it if you skip your regular routine.

Your Pre-Class Warm-Up

Remember, it is important to warm-up before you exercise to prepare your muscles and joints for a strenuous exercise bout. During the warm-up, you need to gradually raise your heart rate. Allow yourself 8 to 10 minutes for a good overall body warm-up. If you are taking an aerobic dance class, it is a good idea to gradually warm-up by walking around the class, stretching slowly and gently before class begins. Afterwards, the following exercises would be good to do as part of your pre-class warm-up.

Stretches and Isolations

Head Isolations

Lift your head up and down. Turn your head to the right, and then to the left. Repeat the set 4 to 8 times.

All photos by Chris Stilians

Rib circles

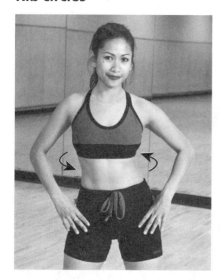

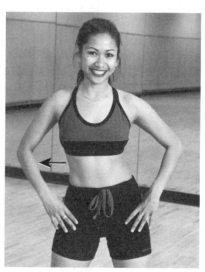

a. Side view: rib isolations forward

Rib isolations

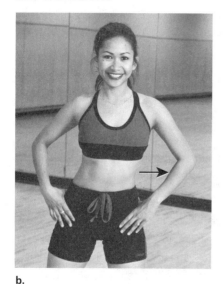

b.

c.

Hip isolations

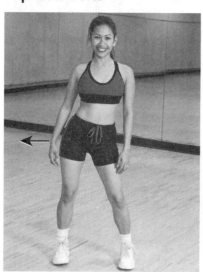

a.

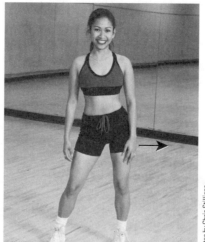

b.

Caution: All head and neck exercises should be performed smoothly and in a relaxed manner. If you allow the neck to arch or roll back, you could put unnecessary tension on the cervical vertebrae.

Shoulder Circles

In a slow, smooth manner, circle your shoulders forward, up, back, and around 8 times. Then, reverse the direction of the roll and repeat it 8 times.

Rib Isolations

While standing with good posture, place your hands on your hips (this helps keep your hips from moving). Move your ribs forward, to the center, to the side, to the center, to the back, to the center, to the other side, and to the center. Repeat by reversing the direction of the rib isolations.

Rib Circles

Perform rib circles the same way as the rib isolations, but in a continuous manner. Do them several times in each direction.

Hip Isolations

While standing with good posture, slightly bend your knees. Now smoothly tilt your pelvis forward, and then backward. Repeat 8 times. Now, tilt your hips and pelvic area to the right, and then the left. Repeat 8 times. Be sure to execute these movements in a smooth, sustained manner.

Hip Circles

While standing with good posture, slightly bend your knees. Smoothly circle your hips forward, to the side, to the back, and to the other side. Continue circling your hips at least 8 times. Now reverse the direction and perform the hip circles the same number of times. Keep your movements smooth and sustained. Jerking movements should be avoided.

All photos by Chris Stillians

Deep Lunge

Begin in a standing position with good posture. With your feet parallel, take a large step forward on one foot. Assume a deep lunge position, with your hands on each side of your knee. The heel of your forward foot must remain on the floor, and the knee should be directly above the foot. Keep your extended back leg straight, with the toes of the foot pushing against the floor. Hold this position for 20 seconds. Now, straighten your forward bent leg and lift the toe up. Gently, without pulling, try to have your head touch your knee. This exercise will stretch your quadriceps, hamstrings, and the Achilles' tendon. Perform the exercise on your other leg. You may want to repeat the entire exercise for each leg.

Side Lunge

Begin in a wide straddle position, with your legs and feet turned out. Bend one knee, and keep the other leg straight. Be sure to keep your knee over your toes and your feet flat while in the lunge position. Lift the toes of the straight leg, and let your hips sink as low as you can to get a nice stretch. Keep your hands on the floor for balance. Hold this position for 15 to 30 seconds, and then perform it on the other side. Repeat the exercise on each side. This exercise stretches the muscles in the inside of your upper leg. These muscles are referred to as your hip flexor muscles.

Hamstring Stretch

While lying on your back, with your feet parallel, bend one leg, keeping your foot

Deep lunge

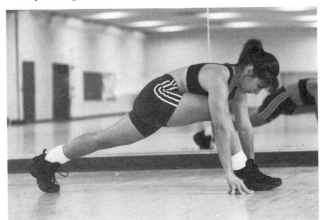

a. Lunge

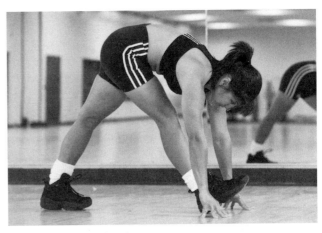

b. Stretch back and flex foot up

Side lunge

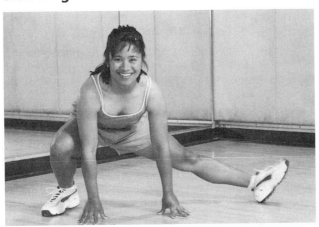

Hamstring stretch

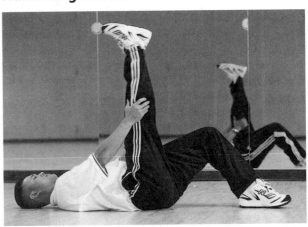

All photos by Chris Stillians

Quadricep stretch

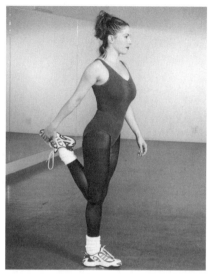

a. Side view

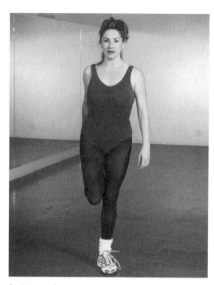

b. Front view

Calf stretches

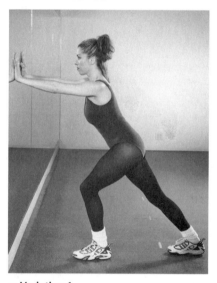

a. Variation 1

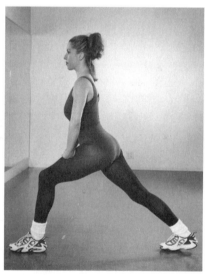

b. Variation 2

Ankle circles while standing

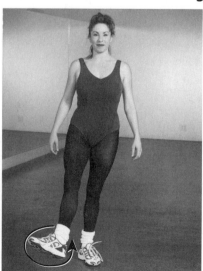

a.

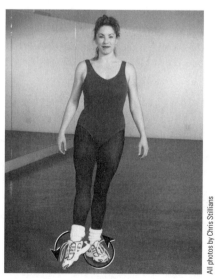

b.

on the ground for support. Lift your other leg up and try to keep the knee straight. Hold the lifted leg under the thigh for a minimum of 15 seconds, preferably for 30 to 60 seconds. This exercise stretches your hamstrings. Repeat on the other side. Perform another set.

Quadriceps Stretch

Stand up with good posture. Keeping your supporting leg slightly bent, grasp your lower leg and gently pull your foot toward your buttocks. Proceed carefully, as this exercise can place stress on your knee joint.

Calf Stretches

Perform either or both of the following calf exercises:

1. Perform a standing lunge by stepping forward with one foot so that your feet are approximately 1 to 2 feet apart. The front leg is bent, while the back leg is straight with the toes facing forward. Hold this position for 20 seconds. Repeat on the other leg. Repeat the set again.

2. Stand facing a wall, approximately 2 feet away from it. Keep your body in a straight line and lunge forward, placing your hands on the wall about shoulder level. In the lunge position, your forward leg is bent, while your back leg is straight. You should feel a stretch in the calf of the straight leg. If you don't, adjust your position until you do. Repeat the exercise again.

Ankle Circles

While standing or sitting, circle your ankles 10 times in each direction. Repeat.

Ankle Raises

From a standing position in good posture, raise yourself up on the balls of your feet. Hold for 4 counts, and then lower yourself back to the floor for 4 counts. Repeat 10 times. Do another set, holding for 2 counts in each position.

Heel Walking

Lift your toes up and walk around the room on your heels. This strengthens your tibialis muscles.

Sitting Straddle Side Stretch

Sit on the floor in a wide straddle position, with your legs straight and your toes pointed. Hold your arms overhead, and stretch to the side. Hold this position for 10 seconds. Repeat on the other side. Repeat the total exercise several times.

    Variation 1: If your knee hurts, bend one leg so the foot faces the body as shown, and stretch over the extended leg (see photo).

    Variation 2: Instead of holding both arms overhead, stretch one arm overhead and stretch the other one toward your toes, as shown in the illustration (see photo).

Sitting Straddle Forward Stretch

Sit on the floor in a wide straddle position. Let gravity pull your torso down, and lean your upper body forward. Be sure to bend from the hips. Hold this position for 10 seconds. Sit up, and repeat the exercise.

Strengthening Exercises

Push-Ups

Perform your maximum number of push-ups. Begin by lying on the floor face down, with your fingers facing forward. Keep your feet together, your abdomen tight and pulled up, your weight on the balls of your feet, and your body in a straight line. Push yourself up until your elbows are straight, but not hyper-extended. Lower your body to the floor halfway (to the point of a 90° angle at the elbows) to perform one push-up. Repeat as many times as you can. This exercise will strengthen your shoulder girdle, pectoralis muscles, biceps, and triceps.

Ankle circles while sitting

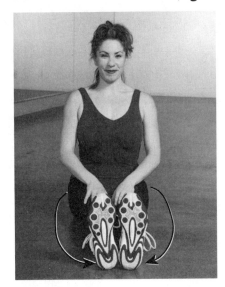

a.

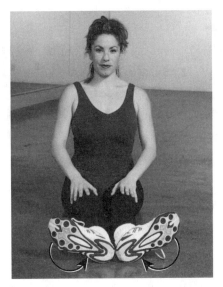

b.

Ankle raises

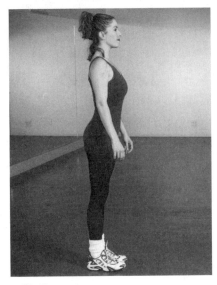

a. Start

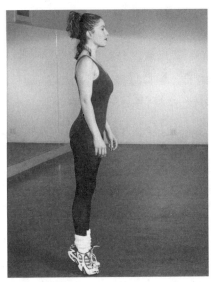

b. Raise on ball of foot

Heel walking

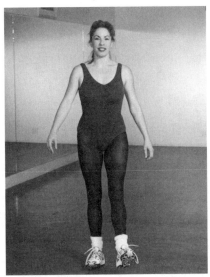

a. Front view (keep toe up)

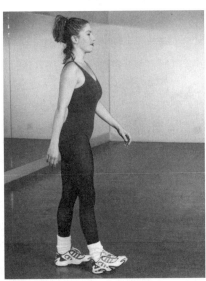

b. Side view

Sitting straddle side stretch

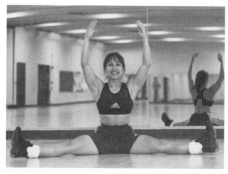
a. Center

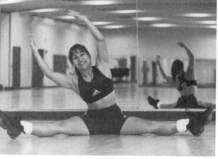
b. Side stretch

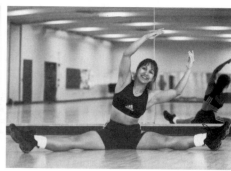
c. Other side stretch

Variation 1: Sitting straddle side stretch while bending one leg

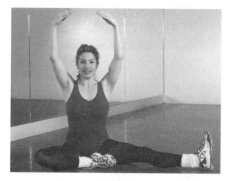
a.

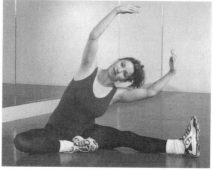
b.

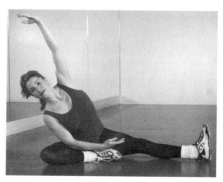
c.

Variation 2: Sitting straddle side stretch

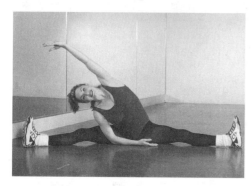

Note: Until you build up the upper body strength to perform full-length push-ups, you may need to perform knee push-ups. The upper body performance is the same as just described; however, the weight of the lower body is supported on the tops of the knee area.

Reverse Push-Ups

This exercise strengthens your triceps muscles. Begin with your weight supported on your hands and feet, and your back parallel to the floor. Your fingers must point toward your heels. Shift most of your weight toward your shoulders. Lower your body halfway to the floor, and then straighten your elbows to return to the starting position. Repeat as many times as possible.

Sitting straddle forward stretch

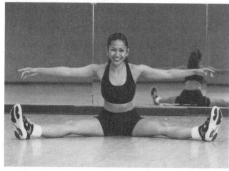
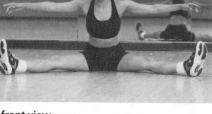
a. front view

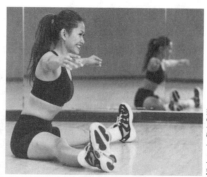
b. side view

Abdominal Curl-Ups

Lie on your back with your knees bent and your feet flat. Place your right hand

Push-ups

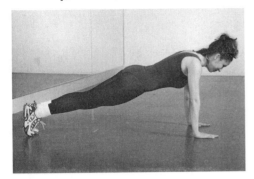 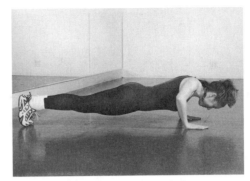

a. Starting position

b.

Push-up variation: bent knee

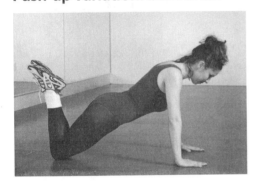 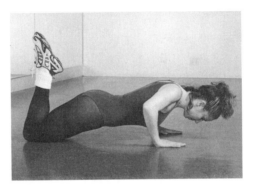

a.

b.

Reverse push-ups

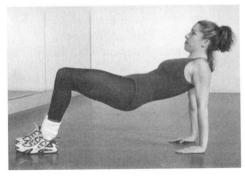 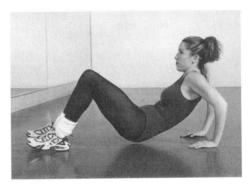

a. Fingertips point toward heels

b.

Abdominal curl-ups

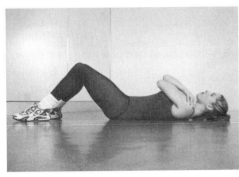 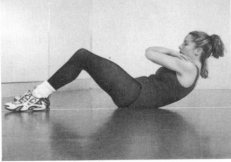

a.

b.

All photos by Chris Stillians

Abdominal curl-ups, front view

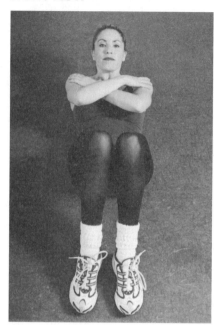

Variation: Abdominal curl-ups, placing arms behind the head

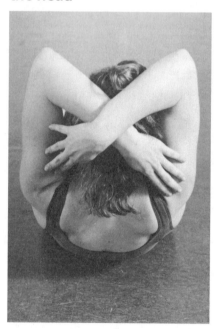

Donkey leg lifts

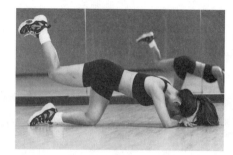

a.

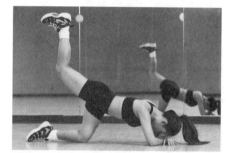

b.

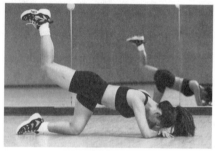

c.

on your left shoulder, and your left hand on your right shoulder. Lift your torso up halfway, keeping your chin tucked toward your chest, and lift your head and shoulders off the floor. (If this hurts your neck, place your arms behind your head, touching opposite shoulders, to cradle the head, keeping your eyes focused above you.) Exhale, contract your abdominal muscles, and press your lower back to the floor as you curl up. Release the contraction. Lower yourself to the floor, being careful not to arch your back. Repeat the curl-up action as many times as you can.

Donkey Leg Lifts

Begin on your hands and knees, with your weight supported on your fore-arms. Keep your head down. Be sure to

Variation: Donkey leg lifts

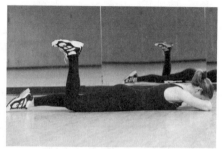

a.

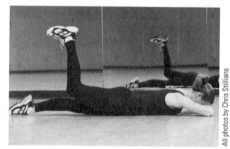

b.

All photos by Chris Stillians

pull your abdominal muscles in tight before you begin. Lift a bent leg up to hip level. Lift your leg in this position several inches, and then lower it to hip level. Keep your hips parallel to the floor, and be sure you don't lean to one side. Repeat this exercise at least 20 times on each leg. This exercise strengthens your gluteal muscles in the buttocks.

Note: A variation of this exercise can be done while you are lying on your stomach (see photo on next page).

Straight Leg Lifts

Begin in the same position described for donkey leg lifts. Extend a straight leg directly in line with the shoulders to 3 to 6 inches below hip level. Now lift your leg up about 6 inches and lower it to the starting position. Never lift the leg above hip level, as that could cause stress on the lower back. Repeat this exercise about 20 times on each leg. Be sure you keep your weight evenly placed, and don't lean to one side. This exercise strengthens your hamstrings.

Side Leg Lifts

Begin by lying on your side. Have the arm closest to the floor support your head

Straight leg lifts

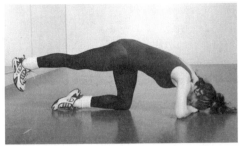

a.

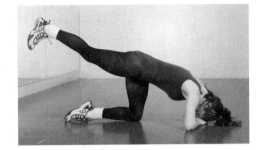

b.

Side leg lifts

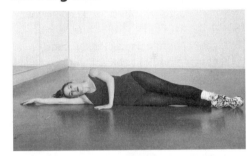

a.

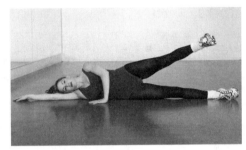

b.

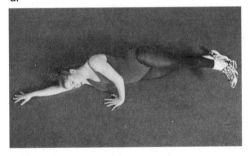

c. Top view

Bent side leg lifts

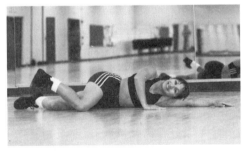

a. Knee down

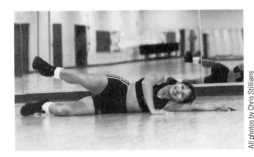

b. Knee lifts

All photos by Chris Stillians

and have the top arm bent in front of your chest, with its palm on the floor. Lift the top leg straight up toward the ceiling, keeping it on a forward diagonal between 30° to 45° from the body (see top view photo). Point the toe slightly toward the floor. Slowly lower the leg. This exercise works the abductor muscles located on the upper outside thigh. Repeat this exercise at least 20 times on each leg.

Bent Side Leg Lifts

Begin by lying on your side. Bend both legs. Bring the top leg up towards the chest, and place the knee and lower leg

Pelvic lifts/buttocks exercises

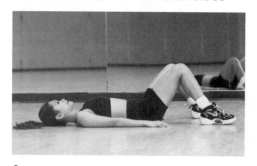

a.

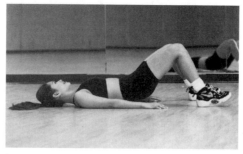

b.

Variation: Pelvic lifts/buttocks exercise

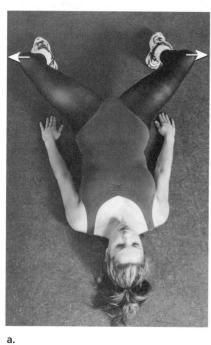

a.

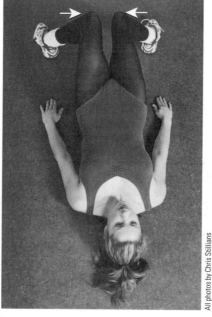

b.

All photos by Chris Stillians

your hands by your sides. Keeping your lower back close to the floor, contract your abdominal muscles and your gluteal muscles to tilt and lift your pelvis approximately 1 to 2 inches toward the ceiling. Keeping your abdominal muscles contracted and your pelvis tilted up, smoothly contract your gluteal muscles. This contraction will gently lift your hips very slightly. Repeat approximately 20 to 30 times.

Caution: Do not lift the lower and middle back off the floor (see photo a).

Variation: Turn your knees and feet out and continue the lifting motion just described another 20 to 30 times in this position. Return your knees to the parallel position. While keeping your pelvis firm and in the position described, bring your knees in toward each other and then out (see photo b).

on the floor for support. Lift the top leg up, hold it there, and then slowly lower it to the floor. Repeat this 20 times on each side. This exercise strengthens the abductor muscles located on the inside of the thigh.

Caution: When performing the side leg lifts or the bent leg lifts, be sure to keep your back straight by contracting your abdominal muscles. In this way, you avoid putting stress on your lower back.

Pelvic Lifts/ Buttocks Exercise

Lie on your back with your knees bent, the soles of your feet on the floor, and

Summary

1. You must commit yourself to a schedule for working out, or you may too easily find excuses why you can't exercise. Set regular times to exercise in your weekly schedule. Once you are in the habit of working out, you will miss it when you can't exercise.

2. Remember, exercising is the best thing you can do for yourself!

3. Perform the exercises described in this chapter. Use the best possible body alignment to gain the most benefit from each exercise and to avoid injuries.

✔ *Checklist for Your Personal Workout*

I plan to workout _____ times per week in an aerobic dance class and _____ times per week _____

Directions: List the repetitions (REPS) and the date you do the following exercises.

Exercise	Date/Reps	Date/Reps	Date/Reps	Date/Reps
Head Isolations				
Shoulder Circles				
Rib Isolations				
Rib Circles				
Hip Isolations				
Hip Circles				
Deep Lunge				
Side Lunge				
Hamstring Stretch				
Quadriceps Stretch				
Calf Stretches				
Ankle Circles				
Ankle Raises				
Heel Walking				
Sitting Straddle Side Stretch				
Sitting Straddle Forward Stretch				
Push-ups				
Reverse Push-ups				
Abdominal Curl-ups				
Donkey Leg Lifts				
Straight Leg Lifts				
Side Leg Lifts				
Bent Side Leg Lifts				
Pelvic Lifts/Buttocks Exercise				

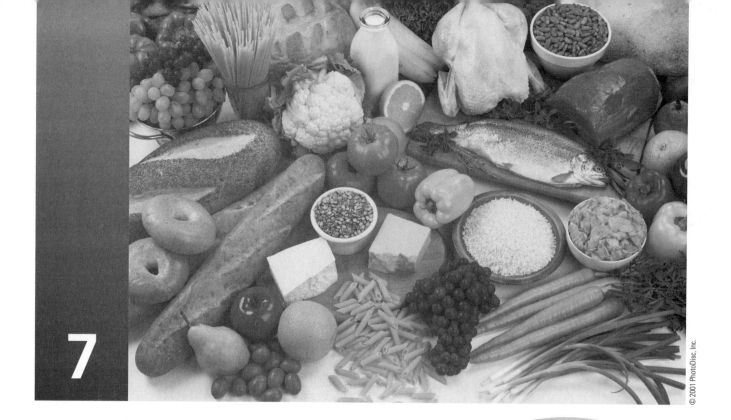

© 2001 PhotoDisc, Inc.

Nutrition

Outline

Basic Nutrition Guidelines
Keep Variety in Your Diet
   Carbohydrates
   Fiber
   Proteins
   Fats
Checklist for Calories Contained
    in Four Food Groups

Water and Hydration
Vitamins and Minerals
Weight Control
Checklist for Calculating
    Desirable Body Weight
Body Composition
Weight Loss
Summary

Basic Nutrition Guidelines

Your body requires a foundation of good nutrition to keep it running at its best. Proper nutrition can be accomplished through good judgment in obtaining the right amount of carbohydrates, proteins, fats, vitamins, minerals, fiber, and water. Good nutrition is important not only in keeping you healthy, strong, and resistant to disease, but also in controlling your weight.

Keep Variety in Your Diet

Hundreds of gimmicky eating plans come and go, but researchers find that eating a variety of foods is the most nutritious means of achieving overall health and longevity. A diet deficient in nutrients increases the risk of developing certain diseases. This is the best reason to avoid fad diets: some can actually be dangerous.

A nutritious diet includes a wide variety of foods from each of the three caloric groups (carbohydrates, proteins, and fats), including sufficient vitamins, minerals, fiber, and water. The American Dietetic Association recommends that your total daily calories be 30 percent fat, 15 percent protein, and 55 percent complex carbohydrates.

Carbohydrates

Carbohydrates, the primary energy source of the body, consist of two kinds: simple and complex. Simple carbohydrates include all forms of sugar, while complex carbohydrates (whole grains, pasta, legumes) serve as a long-acting fuel for the body. The American Dietetic Association and the National Institute of Health recommend that Americans increase their consumption of complex carbohydrates from the meager 25 percent that they've been eating to a level of 55 percent or higher. Carbohydrates provide only four calories per gram and are not as fattening as many people once believed. Carbohydrates are the exclusive fuel for brain function and are stored in the muscles as glycogen, which is used for short-term exercise. Carbohydrates are also "protein sparing," which means that when you consume adequate amounts of carbohydrates, your body is free to use dietary protein for tissue building and repair.

Carbohydrate sources are rich in nutrients, such as B vitamins and iron, as well as fiber. They also help promote a feeling of satiety or fullness. Sources of carbohydrates include milk, breads, cereals, legumes, fruits, and vegetables. Complex carbohydrates consist of a chain of simple sugars and can be recognized as "starchy" rather than sweet. Sugars, such as glucose and sucrose, are carbohydrates, but for the most part are nutrient-poor and contribute empty calories. The average American consumes far too much of this simple sugar: almost 124 pounds per year, much of it hidden in processed foods.

Fiber

Fiber is obtained from whole grains, fruits, and vegetables. Fiber includes both the indigestible, crude type found in wheat bran, and the water-soluble type found in beans and apples. It is important for promoting satiety, regulating bowel function, lowering cholesterol, regulating glucose absorption, and possibly reducing the risk of certain bowel diseases. In general, Americans need to eat about twice as much fiber as they normally do.

Proteins

Proteins are made of amino acids, which are the building blocks of tissues, enzymes, hormones, antibodies, and blood cells. Complete proteins (containing all the essential amino acids) are found in cheese, fish, chicken, milk, meat, and eggs. Vegetables and grains

Checklist for Calories Contained in Four Food Groups

1.	Carbohydrates	4 calories per gram
2.	Fat	9 calories per gram
3.	Protein	4 calories per gram
4.	Alcohol	7 calories per gram

contain incomplete proteins, which can be combined with other types of foods to form complete proteins.

The recommended daily allowance (RDA) for protein is 1 gram of protein for every 2.2 pounds of body weight (.8 grams for every 1 kilogram). For example, a 130-pound woman would require 44 grams; a 154-pound man would require 56 grams. The average American diet contains much more protein than necessary. Although protein contributes only 4 calories per gram, many foods that contain protein also contain fat and, therefore, can increase caloric consumption and contribute to the development of heart disease.

Fats

Fats are an important source of energy and warmth, and are an essential part of cell structure. Some fats are necessary for the absorption of vitamins A, D, and E. These vitamins are also linked to the creation of blood lipids, steroids, cell membranes, and bile.

It is important to limit your intake of saturated fats and fats high in cholesterol, since elevated amounts of these in the bloodstream are associated with heart disease and stroke.

Fats, carbohydrates, and protein make up the caloric values of all foods. While proteins and carbohydrates each contain 4 calories per gram, fats are a calorie-dense food. One gram of fat contains 9 calories. Therefore, fat-laden meals can add a tremendous amount of calories to your daily intake, even though it may appear that you are eating normal quantities of food.

A hamburger fried in grease, with oil-drenched french fries, and a saturated-fat milkshake together contain four times the calories of a meal consisting of fresh salad, applesauce, steamed vegetables, broiled fish, and iced tea with sugar. The typical American diet has too much fat, too many calories, and too few complex carbohydrates.

Water and Hydration

The body generates heat during exercise, which must be dissipated through the evaporation of sweat. Sweat is made up of water, sodium, potassium, and a few other trace elements. For those who participate in aerobic exercise classes, it is very important to replace the water. A good rule of thumb is to drink 8 ounces of water for every hour of aerobics. It is advised to hydrate before, after, and during your exercise class. If you're exercising in extreme heat or high humidity, you will need to drink more. Most dietitians agree that plain, cold water is the best beverage to consume. However, sports drinks are very popular today, and several have recently been developed to meet the needs of the aerobic exercise market. Sports drinks with added electrolytes are most appropriate for strenuous exercise sessions that last close to, or over, 2 hours, such as triathlons, marathons, and various sports games.

Vitamins and Minerals

If you are in good health and eat balanced meals from all four food groups (cereals and grain, meat, dairy, and fruits/vegetables), it's unlikely that you need to supplement your diet with vitamins and minerals. However, many nutritionists recommend a vitamin/mineral supplement if you tend to skip meals occasionally, or if you do not eat as well as you'd like. Mega doses are not necessary; stay within the recommended daily allowances.

Vitamins and minerals are organic compounds that are not made by the body but are required for growth, maintenance, and the repair of cells and tissues. For example, the B-complex vitamins help convert carbohydrate particles into energy molecules known as ATP. Vitamins C and E and the mineral iron are also important for sustaining good health in exercisers. As your exercise workload increases, adherence to a well-balanced diet grows increasingly important.

Weight Control

The first lesson in weight management is how to make proper food choices. However, the importance of an increased level of physical activity as a lifelong tool for weight control is close on its heels, and gaining more impetus every day.

Many factors influence a person's weight fluctuations. We used to think the simple mathematical formula of calorie intake versus calorie output was the chief determinant of body weight. Today, research shows us that the picture is much more complex. Heredity, set-point theory, brown fat deposits, altered basal metabolic rate, and other factors also influence weight control. Heredity, for instance, is definitely gaining speed as a chief indicator of a child's future weight. In studies of identical twins that were raised apart and had very different eating patterns, the twins had similar excessive body fat deposits despite their dissimilar food intake and activity levels.

Set-point theory supports the notion that a body is genetically determined to remain at a certain weight, and that all efforts to increase or decrease that size are unsuccessful in the long run. Supporters of this theory point to the fact that metabolism automatically slows down whenever individuals diet, enabling the set-point weight to remain unchanged.

Brown fat versus yellow fat is another theory that supports a genetic predisposition to obesity. People of normal weight supposedly have more brown fat, a type of capillary-dense fat that surrounds and warms the vital organs and burns deposits of yellow fat as its chief fuel source. Obese individuals, the theory states, did not get their fair share of brown fat deposits at birth, and, as a result, store yellow fat, the visible type that lies under the skin.

However, for those individuals close to their ideal weight, input/output still acts as an important energy equation. The theory can be summarized as follows:

1. ingestion of calories exceeds expenditure of calories = weight gain
2. ingestion of calories is less than expenditure of calories = weight loss
3. ingestion of calories matches expenditure of calories = weight consistency

It is interesting to note that 3,500 calories make up 1 pound of fat. The problem with most weight-loss diets is that they concentrate on the wrong end of the energy equation. Simply decreasing caloric intake without increasing caloric expenditure usually does not result in a permanent loss of fat. You must expend and/or decrease calories by 500 to 1000 per day in order to lose one to two pounds per week. A loss of more than two pounds per week is most likely a loss of body fluid, not fat.

Rapid weight loss followed by periods of rapid weight gain is a common ailment among affluent Western societies. New evidence shows that this yo-yo effect, induced by chronic fad dieting followed by a resumption of normal eating habits, makes an individual fatter over the years. Your total body-fat percentage climbs with successive dieting, because the body grows alert to the "starvation" period while you're dieting and responds by lowering its metabolic rate. This is a survival mechanism, similar to the way hibernating animals store fat for the winter.

The goal of the dieter should be to heighten the body's basal metabolic rate (BMR) by consistent exercise, while maintaining sensible, well-balanced nutritional habits. The basal metabolic rate is the rate at which the body burns energy to conduct all the maintenance activities of daily life. BMR decreases with age and with decreased body surface area. It is slightly slower in women than in men. Exercise can help speed up

---

✓ Checklist for Calculating Desirable Body Weight

To calculate desirable body weight:

1. Determine your present weight. _____ lbs.

2. Determine your percentage of body fat, via skin-fold or other method. _____ %

3. Select the desired body fat. _____ %

4. Subtract the desired body fat from the present body fat. _____ %

5. Multiply the percentage of body fat to be lost by the present weight. _____ lbs.

6. Leads to the desired weight. _____ lbs.

Desired body weight equals the lean body weight divided by the percentage of lean body mass desired.

---

the metabolic rate by increasing the amount of lean muscle in the body.

Body Composition

Body composition refers to the percentage of total body weight that is composed of lean body mass in relation to fat tissue. Body composition cannot be measured on a weight scale, but only through hydrostatic weighing (underwater), electrical impedance (measuring a current through the body), skin-fold calipers (pinching subcutaneous layers), or circumferential measuring (of waist, thigh, and so on). Recommended amounts of fat for young men are 12 to 15 percent; for women, 18 to 22 percent.

The number and size of the fat cells determine the amount of fat on the body. The size of the cells can be stretched through overeating during any phase of a lifetime. One pound of fat stores about 3,500 calories in a form of liquid fat known as triglycerides. Another important fat in the body is cholesterol, which plays a vital role in heart disease, as discussed earlier in the text.

Weight Loss

To lose 1 pound per week, you should have a net deficit of 3,500 calories. Expending more energy and limiting your daily caloric intake to 1,200 to 1,500, depending on your current weight, goal weight, and caloric expenditure, best creates this deficit. Use this formula to determine the number of calories you need to maintain your ideal weight: For women, multiply your ideal weight by 16 if you are very active, 15 if

you are somewhat active, and 14 if you are not very active. (For men, use 17, 16, and 15, respectively.)

For example, if you're a woman weighing 130 pounds and you are not very active, you need 1,820 calories a day (130 × 14). If you increase your activity by adding 1 hour of aerobics each day, you will need 2,080 calories per day to maintain your weight, since the average aerobics class burns 260 calories.

The American Heart Association Dietary Guidelines are listed below for you to read. They suggest a well-balanced diet for Americans to follow for a healthy heart.

American Heart Association Dietary Guidelines At a Glance[1]

1. Achieve an overall healthy eating pattern:

■ Choose an overall balanced diet with foods from all major food groups, emphasizing fruits, vegetables, and grains.

■ Consume a variety of fruits, vegetables, and grain products.

■ Consume at least 5 daily servings of fruits and vegetables.

■ Consume at least 6 daily servings of grain products, including whole grains.

■ Include fat-free and low-fat dairy products, fish, legumes, poultry, and lean meats.

■ Eat at least 2 servings of fish per week.

2. Achieve a healthy body weight:

■ Avoid excess intake of calories.

■ Maintain a level of physical activity that achieves fitness and balances energy

---

[1]© 2000 American Heart Association, Inc.

Food Guide Pyramid: A Guide To Daily Food Choices

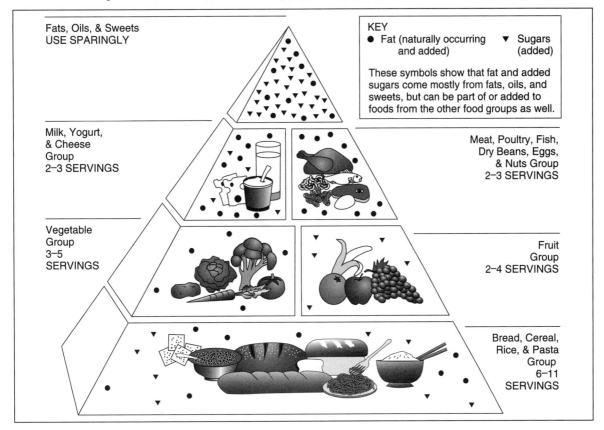

Fats, Oils, & Sweets
USE SPARINGLY

KEY
● Fat (naturally occurring and added)   ▼ Sugars (added)

These symbols show that fat and added sugars come mostly from fats, oils, and sweets, but can be part of or added to foods from the other food groups as well.

Milk, Yogurt, & Cheese Group
2–3 SERVINGS

Meat, Poultry, Fish, Dry Beans, Eggs, & Nuts Group
2–3 SERVINGS

Vegetable Group
3–5 SERVINGS

Fruit Group
2–4 SERVINGS

Bread, Cereal, Rice, & Pasta Group
6–11 SERVINGS

expenditure with caloric intake; for weight reduction, expenditure should exceed intake.

■ Limit foods that are high in calories and/or low in nutritional quality, including those with a high amount of added sugar.

3. Achieve a desirable cholesterol level.

■ Limit foods with a high content of saturated fat and cholesterol. Substitute with grains and unsaturated fat from vegetables, fish, legumes, and nuts.

■ Limit cholesterol to 300 milligrams (mg) a day for the general population, and 200 mg a day for those with heart disease or its risk factors.

■ Limit trans-fatty acids. Trans-fatty acids are found in foods containing partially hydrogenated vegetable oils, such as packaged cookies, crackers, and other baked goods; commercially prepared fried foods; and some margarines.

4. Achieve a desirable blood pressure level.

■ Limit your salt intake to less than 6 grams (2,400 mg sodium) per day, slightly more than one teaspoon a day.

■ If you drink, limit your alcohol consumption to no more than one drink per day for women and two drinks per day for men.

Summary

1. A well-balanced diet includes a wide variety of foods from each of the three caloric groups (carbohydrates, proteins, and fats), including sufficient vitamins, minerals, fiber, and water.

2. Research shows that the proportions of each group that Americans typically eat are not particularly healthful. The typical American diet has far too much fat and protein, and not enough complex carbohydrates.

3. The American Dietetic Association recommends that your total daily calories be 30 percent fat, 15 percent protein, and 55 percent complex carbohydrates.

4. Chronic dieting reduces the amount of lean muscle tissue in the body, which has the net effect of gradually

Nutrition Profile

How to Rate Your Diet

You may want to rate your diet for a few days. Follow these four steps.

Step 1.

Jot down everything you ate yesterday for meals and snacks.	Grams of Fat
Total	

Step 2.

Write down the number of grams of fat in each food you listed.

- Use the Food Guide Pyramid to get an idea of the number of grams of fat to count for the foods you ate.
- Use nutrition labels on the packaged foods you ate to find out the grams of fat they contained.

Step 3.

Answer these questions:

- Did you have the number of servings from the five major food groups that are right for you? (See the previous chart to determine the number of servings that are right for you.)

	Circle the Servings Right for You	Servings You Had
Grain Group Servings	6 7 8 9 10 11	
Vegetable Group Servings	3 4 5	
Fruit Group Servings	2 3 4	
Milk Group Servings	2 3	
Meat Group (ounces)	5 6 7	

How did you do? Not enough? About right?

- Add up your grams of fat listed in Step 2. Did you have more fat than the amount right for you?

	Grams Right for You	Grams You Had
Fat	53 73 93	

How did you do? Too much? About right?

- Do you need to watch the amount of added sugars you eat? See the previous chart to estimate the number of teaspoons of added sugars in your food choices.

	Teaspoons Right for You	Teaspoons You Had
Sugars	6 12 18	

How did you do? Too much? About right?

Step 4.

Decide what changes you can make for a healthier diet. Start by making small changes, like switching to low-fat salad dressings or adding an extra serving of vegetables. Make additional changes gradually until healthy eating becomes a habit.

For More Information
Contact the USDA's Center for Nutrition Policy and Promotion. The address is:
U.S. Department of Agriculture
Center for Nutrition Policy and Promotion
1120 20th St., NW
Suite 200, North Lobby
Washington, D.C. 20036-3475

slowing down your metabolic engine.

5. Regular exercise adds muscle to the body and increases your fat-burning capacity.

6. The body is composed of both lean body mass and fat. Underwater weighing, electrical impedance, skin-fold calipers, or circumferential measurements are ways to measure the amount of fat on the body. The amount of fat recommended should not exceed 18 percent for men and should not exceed 22 percent for women.

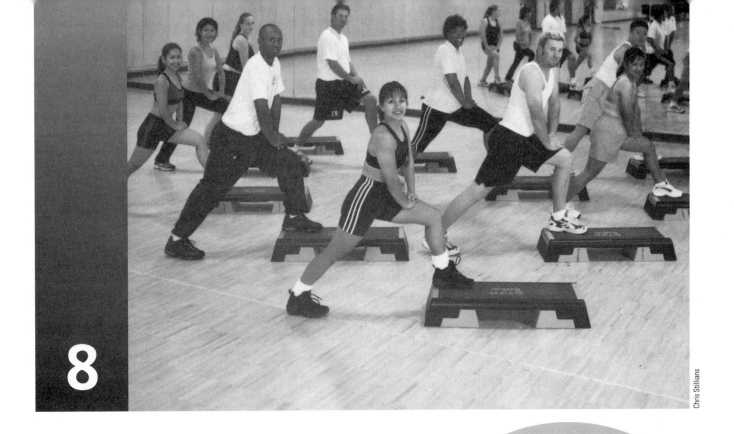

Chris Stillians

8

Injury Prevention

Outline

Prevention of Injury
Pain versus Exercise Discomfort
Treatment for Routine Injuries
Checklist for Treating Injuries
Overuse Injuries
   Plantar Fasciitis
   Achilles' Tendonitis
   Shin Splints
   Stress Reactions and Stress
      Fractures
   Knee Injuries
Common Causes of Aerobics
      Injuries
   Training Errors

Anatomical Problems
Improper Footwear
Training Surfaces
Program Imbalance
Use of Low Weights
Improper Body Alignment
Muscle Imbalance
Nonballistic Stretching
Exercises to Avoid
Heat and Humidity
Exercise-Induced Asthma
Exercise Intolerance
Cardiac Risk Factors
Summary

Prevention of Injury

Aerobic dance exercise has motivated a large segment of the American population toward personal fitness. It will continue to do so as long as the benefits far outweigh any potential for injury.

During the initial thrust of the aerobic dance movement, some early studies revealed injury reports at rates as high as 75 percent for instructors and 45 percent for participants. Most of the injuries were the result of slow-to-heal, nagging overuse injuries, such as shin splints and tendonitis (inflammation of a tendon). In later studies, improper biomechanics and unsafe instructor techniques were cited as the chief reasons for injury. The latest study, conducted in 1987 by the Institute for Aerobics Research and the Aerobics and Fitness Association of America (AFAA), revealed that injury rates had dropped to 35 percent for instructors. Researchers concluded that the use of injury-prevention techniques helped reduce this rate from the earlier reports of 75 percent.

This chapter briefly outlines the significant contributors to aerobic-dance injury, along with recommendations for the safe practice of aerobics.

Pain versus Exercise Discomfort

Staying tuned to your body means being able to tell the difference between the pain of an acute or recent injury and the discomfort of exercise and overuse. Many injuries require immediate medical attention and should not be treated as routine. An injured ankle, for example, often needs to be X-rayed to determine whether there is a fracture. Follow these simple guidelines to determine when to see a doctor. If you answer *yes* to any of the following questions, check with a physician.

1. Is the pain growing worse instead of better, despite rest and initial treatment?

2. Is mobility limited in the injured part?

3. Are you reluctant to place any weight on the limb?

Treatment for Routine Injuries

To treat routine injuries, use the acronym RICE, which stands for:

> Rest
>
> Ice
>
> Compression
>
> Elevation

Under most circumstances, following the four RICE steps will successfully treat common sports injuries. First, if you injure an area, rest it. Do not exercise on it, or the problem will grow worse. You may move the injured part without placing weight on it, in order to maintain circulation and promote healing to the area.

Second, apply ice to the injured part for 10 to 15 minutes at a time, as soon as possible after the injury. Slowly massage the area with an ice cube, but protect the skin with a thin sheet. This constricts the blood vessels, reduces swelling, and numbs the area for a short while.

Next, securely wrap the area with an elastic bandage, but not so tightly that you cut off all circulation. Following an

Checklist for Treating Injuries

Rest: Refrain from any further activity.

Ice: Apply ice massage for 10 to 15 minutes as soon as possible after injury.

Compression: Wrap affected area in elastic bandage.

Elevation: Keep the area above heart level if possible.

ice massage, circulation increases. Compressing the injured area helps to prevent excessive swelling and further damage in the area. Finally, elevate the injured area above heart level to prevent excessive swelling. This promotes healing as well.

Overuse Injuries

Overuse injuries result from repeated stress placed on the body as a result of too much activity too soon. Prevention is the best treatment, since overuse injuries are tough to completely heal. Excessive exercise causes a breakdown of cells in the muscles, tendons, bones, and cartilage. Damage to tissues causes swelling and pain. Pain usually convinces you to rest, which allows time for repair and growth of new cells. If you exercise despite painful warnings, further cell damage occurs, leading to tendonitis and muscle strains. Stress reactions in the lower leg bones (tibia and fibula) or the bones of the feet can lead to tiny, painful stress fractures if the overuse continues unchecked.

Plantar Fasciitis

Plantar fasciitis causes pain or burning on the sole of the foot, midfoot to heel. This injury occurs when the plantar fascia ligament, which connects the heel to the ball of the foot, is overstretched. Commonly called a sprained arch, this injury often results from a pronated (flattening of the arch) foot, which pulls on the fascia or sheath covering the muscle.

Treatment often starts with a good arch support prescribed by a foot specialist (podiatrist). It is also often necessary to apply an ice massage to the area after a workout.

Achilles' Tendonitis

This fairly common injury results in pain and stiffness in the heel cord, which connects the calf muscle to the heel bone.

Wearing inadequate shoes, running on hard surfaces, doing improper warm-ups, and doing insufficient stretching are some causes of Achilles' tendonitis.

Treatment consists of RICE (rest, ice, compression, and elevation), as described earlier in the chapter. Once healing has occurred, make sure you sufficiently stretch the tendon with a good calf stretch before and after your workout.

Shin Splints

This is a catch-all term describing any discomfort in the front lower leg, sometimes involving muscles and fascia, and sometimes involving bone inflammation. Shin splints are fairly common among beginners, those exercising on concrete floors, or those without well-cushioned shoes.

Preventing shin splints is certainly preferable to treating them, since they tend to take several weeks or months to disappear. Exercise only on well-cushioned floors and wear appropriate aerobics shoes. Also try to perform shin-strengthening exercises, such as lifting the toes toward the knee with a weight wrapped around the forefoot. In cases of painful shin splints, RICE should give you relief.

Stress Reactions and Stress Fractures

Stress reactions or fractures may be confused with shin splints when they occur in the lower leg. Among aerobics enthusiasts, they are more commonly found in the feet. Stress reactions are a warning that the body is a victim of the overuse syndrome and that it's time to slow down, rest, and repair. Stress reactions that are ignored progress into full fractures.

If diagnosed by a bone scan, stress fractures require medical treatment.

Knee Injuries

Knee injuries in aerobics are usually related to either: (1) compression forces from jumping, resulting in a chronic ache, known as chrondomalacia; or (2) torque forces, resulting in a twisting of the knee, with injury to the ligaments or tendons. Proper alignment of the knees directly over the toes (never over-reaching them) is very important in preventing knee ligament strains.

RICE may help initially, but knees are very vulnerable to injury, so proceed with caution. Knee injuries tend to make return visits. Check the soles of your shoes to make sure they are not overly worn. Try strengthening all the muscle groups that support and stabilize the knee. Working with an athletic trainer or physical therapist can improve the function and stability of your knees.

Common Causes of Aerobics Injuries

Training Errors

Doing too much too soon is a common training error. Suddenly increasing your training means that there is inadequate time for tissues to adapt to the challenging workload.

Do no more than 15 to 20 minutes of aerobics for the first few weeks, and then advance to 30 minutes after two months. Advance gradually after that, as long as there are no signs of injury.

The beginner should take no more than six classes per week. The highly conditioned participant may safely take up to twelve classes per week.

Anatomical Problems

Anatomical problems include such things as having one leg be longer than the other (which may throw off gait and alignment), knock-knees, fallen arches, rigid foot (very high arch), muscle imbalances, scoliosis or curved spine, pronated feet, and obesity.

Improper Footwear

Supportive footwear is absolutely necessary in aerobic exercise classes to decrease the amount of shock transmitted up the body. The impact from foot strike can be two to three times greater without shock-absorbing shoes. Poor-fitting or inappropriate shoes can also

cause problems. Shoes that compact easily or lose their cushioning with use can cause stress injuries. Adequate lateral support in shoes is also very important in reducing the amount of shock.

Sometimes arch supports recommended by a sports podiatrist can reduce problems such as arch fatigue or excessive pronation (foot rolling to the inside).

Training Surfaces

High-impact aerobic exercise produces a percussive, vertical impact of foot strike, which leads to overuse injuries of the lower extremities. Impact is a product of force (how hard you work or how high you pick your feet up) times repetition.

The best types of floor surfaces are those which provide adequate cushioning, yet maintain stability. Floors associated with the highest rates of injury include concrete, linoleum, and carpet over concrete. Optimal floors for aerobic dance are the following:

1. suspended wood

2. coiled-spring wood

3. shock-absorbing mats or special vinyl flooring

4. carpet over mats or over a suspended floor or rubber flooring

Program Imbalance

Aerobic workouts that are not complemented with programs designed to improve flexibility, muscular endurance, muscular strength, coordination, agility, and balance can create an overall imbalance problem. Even periods of rest are considered essential to an exercise program. All of these factors are part of total fitness.

Use of Low Weights

Low weights can act as an added challenge for the cardiovascular and musculoskeletal systems once training gains start to plateau. But safe use of the weights is essential in order to avoid injury to the joints, tendons, and muscles. (Read the following chapter, "Low-Impact Aerobics" for advice on the use of low weights.)

Improper Body Alignment

Proper body alignment during aerobic exercise can keep participants injury-free, with no back discomfort or knee pain. It is important to start with proper posture, which means keeping the planes of the body in a neutral midpoint. The trunk must be balanced in a neutral position, held in place by strong abdominal muscles in the front, and by strong gluteals, hamstrings, and lower back muscles posteriorly. The knees must be over the toes, with the weight forward on the metatarsals.

You risk fatiguing your muscles faster and injuring your joints if your body is not aligned correctly. Ankles, knees, hips, torso, shoulders, neck, and head need to line up in proper alignment—think of your body as a set of boxes stacked one on top of the other.

When you stand, the patella (kneecap) and the toes should be facing the same direction. When lunging, keep the knees and toes in the same direction, and make sure the knees never extend beyond the toes, laterally or medially.

Muscle Imbalance

Muscles oppose each other to move each of the body's levers at the joints. For example, the biceps contract, flexing the forearm, while their opposing muscles, the triceps, relax and stretch. When the triceps contract, the forearm is extended, and this time, the biceps stretch. When muscles are out of balance, or when one muscle is much stronger than its opposing muscle, injury is more likely to happen.

Muscle groups that come into play during aerobic exercise routines include:

1. adductors and abductors
2. quadriceps and hamstrings
3. gastrocnemius and tibialis anterior
4. abdominals and erector spinae
5. biceps and triceps
6. pectorals and rhomboids, trapezius

Whenever a muscle or muscle group is strengthened, it should also be stretched. Otherwise, it will overpower its opposing muscle. For example, running can strengthen both quadriceps and hamstring muscles. If, after a run, an individual stretches the quadriceps, but consistently fails to stretch the hamstrings, a serious imbalance occurs. The hamstring grows progressively tighter and shorter, pulling the pelvis out of alignment and creating low back discomfort. Of course, stretching alone does not prevent serious strength imbalances. Attention should also be paid to balancing the strength-training regimen. However, it is important that opposing muscle groups be stretched to the point of mild tension and held for a minimum of 20 seconds during cool-down.

Nonballistic Stretching

Ballistic stretching is not recommended during warm-up or cool-down. As discussed earlier, ballistic or bouncing stretches are those that elicit the stretch reflex, a protective reflex of the neuromuscular system, similar to a knee jerk. It prevents the muscle from overstretching by actually contracting it. Some exercise professionals believe that static, slow stretches (nonballistic) elongate the muscle, helping to rid the fibers of toxic byproducts of metabolism, such as lactic acid. Stretch to the point of mild tension, not pain. Go only as far as you can comfortably tolerate.

Exercises to Avoid

The following exercises place undue stress on the joints, seriously overstretch ligaments, and create torque-like or twisting forces to vertebrae and joints throughout the body:

1. back arching or hyper-extension
2. hurdler's stretch
3. yoga plough
4. straight leg lifts
5. windmill toe touches
6. deep knee bends
7. full sit-ups
8. rapid side-to-side twisting
9. side leg swings on hands and knees

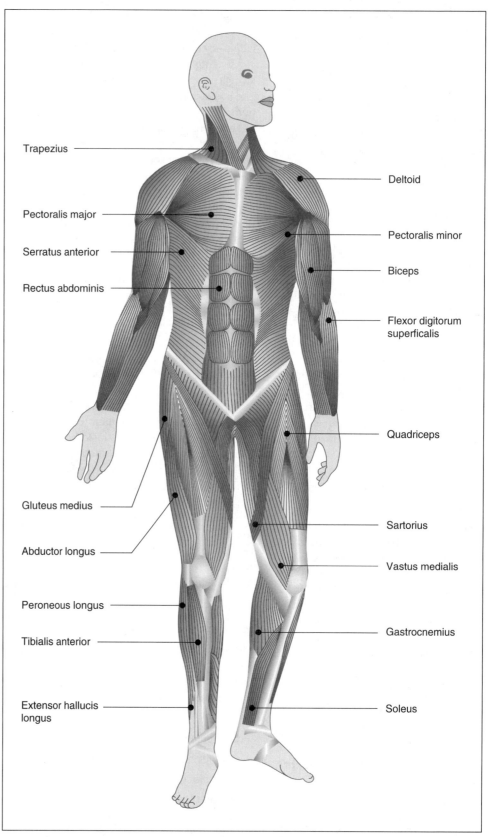

Trapezius

Deltoid

Pectoralis major

Pectoralis minor

Serratus anterior

Biceps

Rectus abdominis

Flexor digitorum
superficalis

Quadriceps

Gluteus medius

Sartorius

Abductor longus

Vastus medialis

Peroneous longus

Gastrocnemius

Tibialis anterior

Extensor hallucis
longus

Soleus

Muscle groups, front view

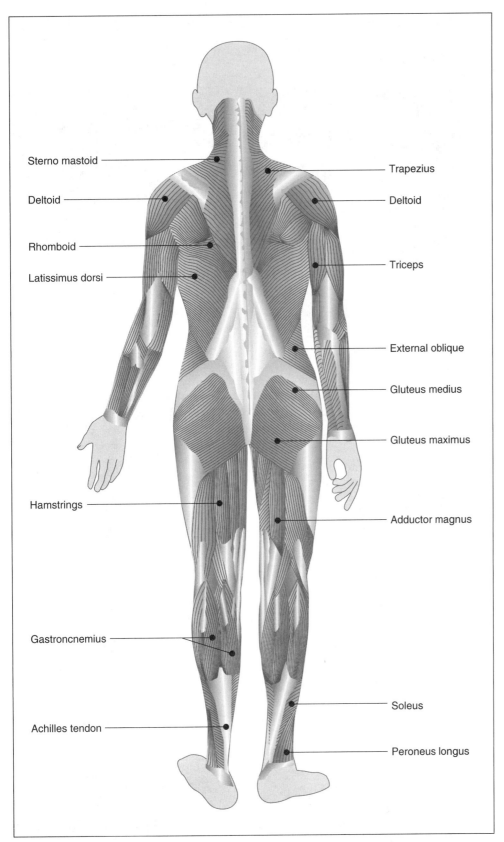

Sterno mastoid

Deltoid

Rhomboid

Latissimus dorsi

Hamstrings

Gastroncnemius

Achilles tendon

Trapezius

Deltoid

Triceps

External oblique

Gluteus medius

Gluteus maximus

Adductor magnus

Soleus

Peroneus longus

Muscle groups, back view

**Exercises to avoid:
Back arching or
hyperextension of the neck**

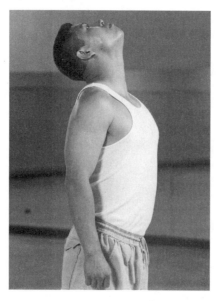

Yoga plough

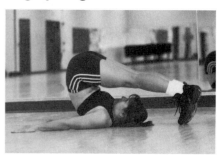

Hurdler's stretch

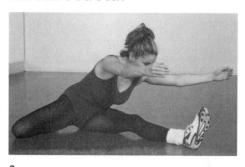

a.

b. Top view; variation

Straight leg lifts

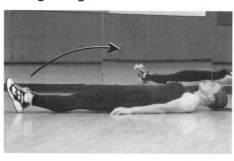

a.

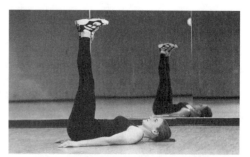

b.

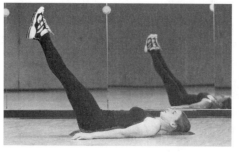

c.

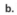
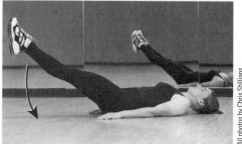

d.

Exercises to avoid:
Windmill toe touches

Deep knee bends

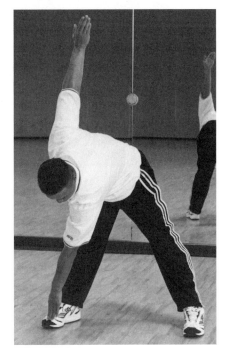

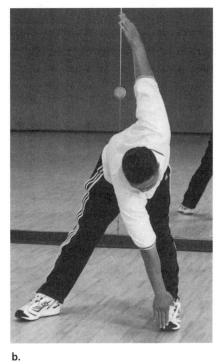

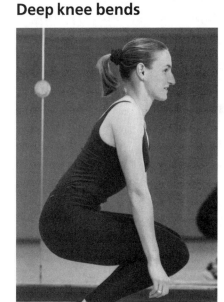

a.

b.

Full sit-ups

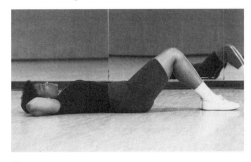

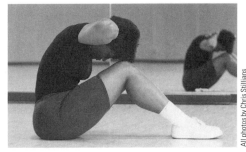

All photos by Chris Stillians

a.

b.

Heat and Humidity

A major byproduct of muscular work is heat, which raises the body's core temperature. The circulating blood carries this heat to the surface of the skin, where it is released via the opening of pores and the evaporation of sweat. The sweat produced during 1 to 2 hours of exercise consists primarily of water, along with some minor amounts of sodium, urea, uric acid, and amino acids.

Drinking 8 ounces of water for every 20 minutes of exercise is a good rule of thumb for rehydration. Water is the chief regulatory element for keeping your body's aerobic engine cool.

Never exercise in clothing that inhibits evaporation of sweat from the body (materials such as nylon and non-permeable plastic wraps); otherwise, serious heat injury can result.

On hot and humid days, sweat may not have a chance to evaporate, causing your body to retain heat and raise your core temperature. Lower the intensity of exercise during these periods so that heat injury is not risked.

**Exercises to avoid:
Rapid side-to-side twisting**

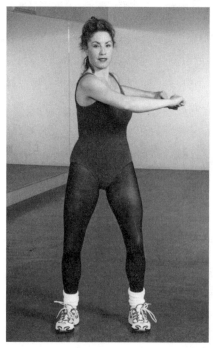

a.

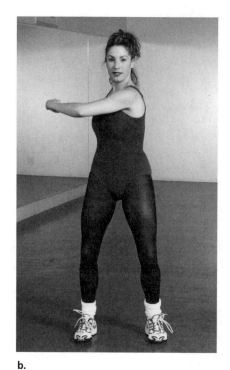

b.

Side leg swings on hands and knees

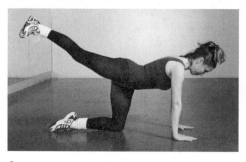

a.

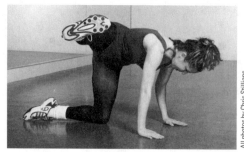

b.

All photos by Chris Stillians

Exercise-Induced Asthma

This is a type of allergic response to exercise, characterized by wheezing and difficulty in breathing. Inhalant medication can alleviate the symptoms. Check with a physician before proceeding with exercise should these symptoms arise.

Exercise Intolerance

If you have any of the following abnormal responses to exercise, you need to check with a physician before continuing the exercise program. These symptoms could indicate cardiovascular disease or an impending heart attack or stroke:

1. light-headedness
2. dizziness
3. ringing in ears
4. excessive shortness of breath
5. chest pain, heaviness, or burning
6. jaw pain
7. arm pain, numbness, or tingling
8. nausea or vomiting
9. irregular pulse or sudden palpitations

10. fever

11. hives, swelling, or itching

12. severe aches and pains in a particular area of the body

If any of the above conditions develop while exercising, stop immediately, cool down if possible, and seek medical attention.

Cardiac Risk Factors

The following list of risk factors contribute to the incidence of heart disease:

Advanced age: Risk increases over age 50.

Male gender: Risk is higher in males than in females.

High blood pressure: A chief contributor of heart attacks. The upper limit for a young adult is 140/90; lower limit is 70/50. Normal range is around 120/80.

Family history of heart problems: A positive history means frequent check-ups.

Sedentary lifestyle: Inactivity increases cholesterol and contributes to obesity.

Smoker: Increases the risk of heart disease fourfold.

Diabetic: Risk is greater for insulin-dependent diabetes.

Elevated cholesterol and triglyceride levels in the blood: These contribute to heart disease and stroke.

If you have a history of cardiovascular disease, or any medical condition, you should get medical clearance before engaging in vigorous aerobic exercise. Exercise can be an excellent therapeutic tool in the treatment of diabetes, obesity, cardiovascular disease, stress disorders, and musculoskeletal limitations, when supervised and engaged in properly.

Summary

1. The most common types of injuries in aerobic dance are known as overuse injuries, which result from too much stress over too short a period of time. Cellular damage to muscles, bones, and other tissues requires time for repair and the growth of new cells. Exercising despite painful warnings can lead to further damage.

2. A standard initial treatment for minor sports injuries consists of rest, ice, compression, and elevation, commonly called RICE. Ice should be applied to the injured part for at least 10 to 15 minutes, followed by a secure wrap and elevation.

3. Common overuse injuries include inflammation of the sole of the foot (plantar fasciitis) and the Achilles' tendon, shin splints, stress reactions and fractures, and knee injuries.

4. Attention should be paid to balancing overall fitness with programs for flexibility, muscular endurance, strength, coordination, agility, and balance. Opposing muscles should be balanced in strength and flexibility so that injuries and tears are avoided.

5. Proper body alignment during aerobic exercise is an essential component of injury prevention.

6. Certain movements should be avoided altogether in a safe aerobics program. These include ballistic or bouncing stretches during warm-up and cool-down, and any exercises that place undue stress on the joints or ligaments.

7. An aerobic exercise enthusiast should be in tune with his or her body and learn to recognize any sign of exercise intolerance, such as overheating, difficulty in breathing, light-headedness, or pain.

8. Anyone with a history of medical problems or physical limitations should seek a physician's approval before beginning a vigorous aerobics program.

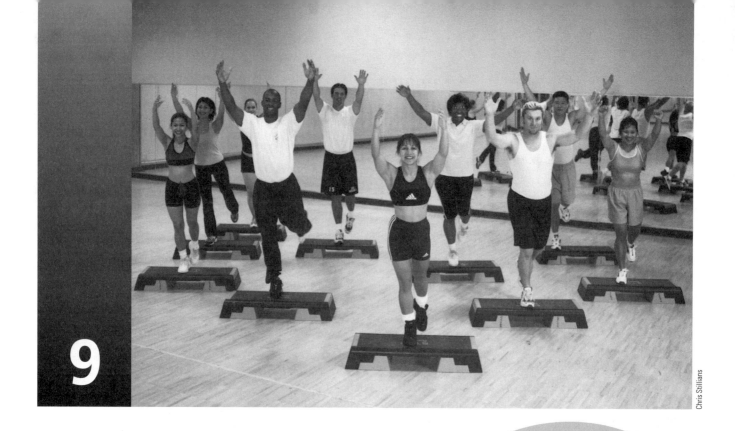

Chris Stillians

Low-Impact Aerobics

Outline

Definition

Impact and Injuries

Protecting the Knees

Checklist for Knee Protection

Low-Back Precautions

The Question of Weights

When Not to Use Weights

Low-Impact versus Low-Intensity

Aqua Aerobics Exercise

Body Sculpting

Other Low-Impact Alternatives

Benefits

Summary

Low impact aerobics stresses vigorous upper body movement, while focusing on smooth transitions

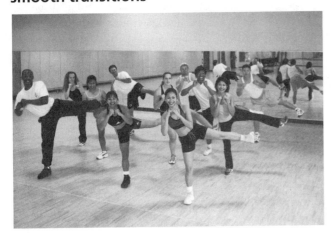

Kick boxing class

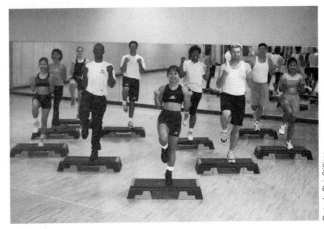

Step aerobics class

Photos by Chris Stillians

Definition

Low-impact aerobics is a form of aerobic exercise that is perfect for anyone who wants to avoid the jumping and jarring movements performed in traditional high-impact classes. The basic rule in low-impact aerobics is to keep one foot on the floor at all times while performing vigorous upper body moves. There is, however, a lot more to low-impact aerobics than simply "grounding" a high-impact class. Instructors must try to make their students mentally alert as to how their bodies are moving. They not only have to concentrate on the intensity of a movement, but they also have to focus on a full range of motion and smooth transitions. The careful patterning and sequencing of a class are instrumental in achieving the desired cardiovascular training effects. Some experts say that low-impact is not so much a new trend as it is simply a new name. Those who have conducted classes for over 15 years find it interesting to watch the return of dance-like movements, which are replacing the jumping and hopping of traditional aerobics.

The following guidelines should help make a low-impact class safe, yet enjoyable.

Impact and Injuries

Whenever the feet come into contact with the floor, there is an impact. Frequent, high-impact movements that are not done safely may lead to injuries. Injuries from high-impact aerobics are generally overuse injuries relating to compression or impact trauma. As discussed in the previous chapter, they include shin splints, stress reactions, stress fractures, plantar fasciitis, tendonitis, and so on. Low-impact aerobics emerged with the goal of reducing the impact of jumping and running-in-place movements.

Has the injury rate actually decreased? It's likely that injuries to the lower extremities have decreased, and that the sites of injuries have shifted from shins, Achilles' tendons, and feet in high-impact aerobics to knees, lower backs, shoulders, and arms in the low-impact variety. Before any definite conclusions can be made regarding the safety of low-impact aerobics, research needs to be done.

In low-impact aerobics, as in high-impact classes, you need to pay attention to using proper footwear and resilient floor surfaces. Floors should be either carpeted over mats, highly stable mats, or spring or suspension wood floors. Shoes, once again, are important.

The quick side-to-side movements you make during low-impact aerobics require extensive lateral support in an appropriate shoe.

However, when all factors are taken into account, the instructor's technique seems to be the single most important consideration in injury prevention. The best pair of shoes and the latest, safest floor won't protect you from improper biomechanical (body position) form, or dangerous exercises.

Protecting the Knees

The quick, lateral movements in a low-impact class can endanger the knees. Be aware of your center of gravity (in the center of your hips), and keep it balanced over the midfoot. Make sure the knees never overshoot the toes when you do side lunges. This action over-stretches knee ligaments and makes the joint unstable. Keep your knees facing the same direction as the lower leg and toes when you do side lunges. Whenever the knee points in one direction and the leg twists in the opposite direction, a force known as torque creates excessive stress on the knee joint. Be sure to pick your feet up—don't let the toes drag against the floor when switching directions. Also, try to build the strength in your quadriceps (front thigh muscles) and hamstrings for added protection. Don't expect your knees to compensate for weak leg muscles.

Low-Back Precautions

Make sure you don't arch your back when you raise your arms overhead, and don't lean forward without supporting your upper body weight. Slow down the movements and avoid hyper-extending the shoulder joint. When standing, the best way to avoid arching the back is to make sure your abdominal muscles are contracted, pelvis is tucked, rib cage is lifted, and knees are slightly bent.

The Question of Weights

You may want to try using hand-held or wrist weights in class. Some instructors feel that weights give an added boost to the cardiovascular challenge in a class, once individuals have reached such a high level of conditioning that it's difficult for them to attain their target heart rate. However, research indicates that weights under two pounds do not significantly contribute to the cardiovascular conditioning effect. If your arms are lacking any muscular definition or tone, weights may put you on the road to minor gains in muscular endurance and strength. On the whole, most instructors have a policy of using weights during the conditioning portion of a class, but never during the aerobics portion. Some instructors allow the use of hand-held or attached-wrist low weights (2 to 3 pounds) during the aerobic portion of class, but not ankle weights. In so doing, they are consistent with the AFAA Standards and Guidelines for Weighted Workouts. Heavier weights are to be used in a stationary position. Therefore, ankle weights may be used for lower body strengthening in a stationary position.

Keep the movements controlled, smooth, and within the normal range of motion for the joint. Rapid jerking movements with weights can cause problems in the elbow joint, forearms, shoulders, and arm muscles. Again, make sure you

Checklist for Knee Protection

1. When standing, never overextend the knees beyond the toes.

2. Make sure the knee, ankle, and mid-foot are in straight alignment.

3. Never bring the hips below the level of the knees in a working squat or lunge.

are not hyperextending or bending the joint past its normal anatomical position. Also, don't snap the joint. Tendons in the wrist and forearms can be inflamed due to overuse of weak muscles and over-gripping of low weights. Don't let the arm snap up and roll backward. The head of the bicep muscle can become seriously inflamed, requiring about 4 to 6 weeks of rest, plus physical therapy and medical treatment.

Weights are for non-beginners only. People who can perform sixteen repetitions without fatigue are probably ready for weights. Start with the smallest weight (1 pound), then gradually progress, but do not exceed 3 pounds during aerobic work. Ankle weights should only be used during strengthening exercises for the lower body, and never during aerobics. Remember to keep weights off during the warm-up and cool-down portions of class. Joints, tendons, and muscles need at least a 10-minute warm-up period to prepare for the added stress of weights.

Beginners tend to grip the hand weights too tightly and actually impair blood flow in the arms, owing to a continuous isometric contraction. This action can raise blood pressure to serious levels. People with high blood pressure or a history of stroke or heart disease should consult their physicians prior to exercising with weights. If joint soreness or muscular pain develops, stop using weights and rest.

Let your heart rate monitor whether you should add or subtract weights. Your heart rate will climb whenever additional weight is added.

When Not to Use Weights

1. Do not use weights during the pre-aerobic warm-up or post-aerobic cool-down.

2. Do not use hand-held or ankle weights while performing high-impact movements.

Proper use of weights

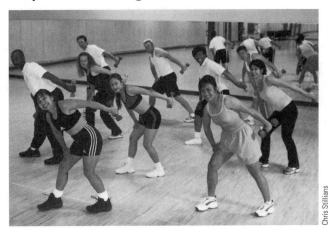

Chris Stillians

3. Do not use weights on a limb that has been injured unless it has been recommended and supervised by a physician.

Low-Impact versus Low-Intensity

Low-impact often gets confused with low-intensity. Low-impact refers to a reduced-impact stress on the feet, legs, knees, and hips, not to a lower intensity. Low-intensity refers to a reduced workload, or working at a lower heart rate. There are beginner, intermediate, and advanced classes for people at various levels of fitness. You can lower the intensity of a low-impact class by keeping arm movements below shoulder height until you gradually gain strength. Instead of performing high-stepping movements, simply march in place. Don't raise the knees quite as high. Avoid complex patterns if you're a beginner. You'll be ready to join in again if you can carry on a brief conversation comfortably, or if you remain at your target heart rate while working.

Aqua Aerobics Exercise

While aqua aerobics/water exercise has been around for many years, according to the Aquatic Exercise Association (AEA), water aerobics is a relative newcomer to the fitness scene. It is gaining popularity because of its nonstressful, nonpercussive style. Jane Katz, Ed.D., author of the "The New W.E.T. Workout Water Exercise Techniques for Strengthening, Toning,

Aqua aerobics water exercise

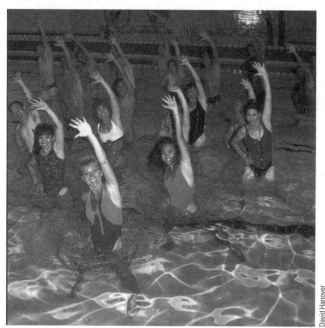

David Hanover

Body sculpting class

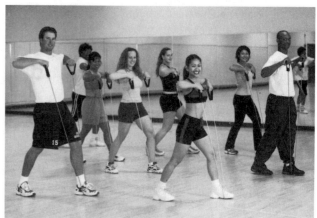

Chris Stillians

and Lifetime Fitness" (1996), advocates water aerobics for all individuals, but finds it especially well-suited for overweight individuals. The buoyancy and resistance of water make a 150-pound person weigh only 15 pounds. Water aerobics is usually done in chest-deep water; swimming is not usually part of the routine. Classes are geared to all types of people: rehabilitating athletes, seniors, pregnant women, arthritis patients, and people who simply love the water. For more information on water aerobics, read *Aqua Aerobics Today* by Carole Casten, Ph.D., Wadsworth Publishing Company.

Body Sculpting

A variation of the low-impact class is what is often titled a *body sculpting class.* This class usually begins with a low-impact aerobic warm-up activity, followed by a variety of exercises using hand-held weights and/or exercise resistance bands. Often these exercises are alternated with low-impact aerobic movements. This class has gained in popularity for individuals who want to take a combined strength and aerobic endurance class in a limited time frame of approximately 1 to 1 1/2 hours.

Other Low-Impact Alternatives

Many health clubs offer classes in Pilates, Yoga, and Power Yoga. These classes provide alternative low-impact fitness activities that include strength, endurance, and stretching activities.

Benefits

The benefits of a low-impact class are identical to those of any aerobic exercise-training program. The benefits include:

1. lowered resting heart rate

2. lowered resting blood pressure

3. reduced triglycerides

4. increased HDL cholesterol (the protective type of cholesterol)

5. enhanced basal metabolic rate

6. less overall body fat

7. improved cardiopulmonary efficiency

8. improved ability to cope with stress

9. preferred form of aerobics after returning from an injury

However, just like with traditional aerobics, you achieve benefits only if you exercise with sufficient frequency, duration, and intensity. The aerobic portion of class must be at least 20 minutes long, with heart rates in the training heart rate range, and you must attend class (or get the equivalent workout outside of class) at least three or four times per week.

It is premature to state whether there will be less injuries in low-impact aerobics compared with traditional aerobics. We may just see a shift in injuries from shins and feet to shoulders and backs. Any part of the body can be subjected to overuse injuries. Injury usually results from too much, too soon. However, compression or impact trauma is not the only cause of overuse injuries. Therefore, use common sense to pace yourself.

Summary

1. Low-impact aerobics can be an enjoyable form of exercise and a welcome change from high-impact classes.

2. Low-impact aerobics is a relative newcomer to the aerobic field, and is welcomed by those who wish to avoid the jumping in a high-impact class. It consists of vigorous upper body moves, coupled with leg movements that allow you to keep one foot on the floor at all times.

3. It is important to protect the knees when performing the quick lateral movements in a low-impact class. Try to avoid extending the knee beyond the toes. Also try to keep the knee and the foot pointing in the same direction whenever switching back and forth quickly.

4. Hand-held weights can add a challenge to the cardiovascular system for advanced exercisers. Some precautions should be taken when working with weights. Make sure your back does not arch when your arms are raised overhead, and definitely avoid rapid, jerking movements. Work the weights with a slow, controlled style.

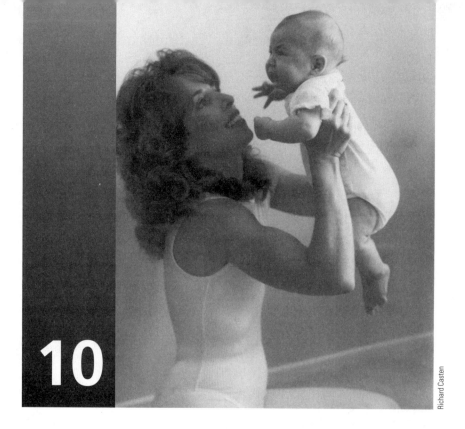

Pregnancy and Aerobic Dance Exercise

Outline

Value
Special Precautions
  Medical Clearance
  Fluids
  Warning Signs that Indicate
    the Need to Stop Exercising
Modifications to an Aerobic
    Exercise Program
  Warm-up
  Cardiovascular Work
  Floor Work
  Cool-Down Stretches
Special Exercises

Low-Impact Movement
  Kegel Exercises
  Standing Work
Controversial Exercises
Exercises to Avoid
  High Knee Lifts
  Quick Lateral Movements
  High-Impact Jumping and
    Jarring
  Weights
  Traditional Rejects
  Prone Position
Summary

Richard Casten

10

Value

Pregnancy and aerobic dance exercise can be safe partners. Aerobic dance can have a healthy and positive effect on a mom-to-be, and help her with a rapid recovery during the post-partum period. A prenatal class should be taught by a trained professional to meet the physical and emotional needs of the pregnant exerciser. Classes offered in conjunction with childbirth education are among the most conscientious programs.

Exercise does not necessarily decrease labor time or insure a healthier baby. However, it does directly provide quite a few benefits to the mother, and indirectly to the developing fetus. Research supports the finding that, through aerobics, the exercising mother-to-be can maintain her own cardiovascular fitness, musculoskeletal strength, and flexibility. Benefits to the fetus are less well defined. However, sufficient data supports the finding that the fetus is not endangered during a pregnant woman's consistent exercise for periods of 15 minutes or less when her heart rate is no higher than 140 beats per minute. As the pregnancy advances, the woman and her physician should continue to evaluate her tolerance to aerobic exercise, and whether or not she should exercise to full term.

Special Precautions

Medical Clearance

Pregnant women should seek a physician's clearance before beginning or altering an exercise program.

Fluids

Pregnant women should be encouraged to drink freely before, during, and after a workout to avoid dehydration. Exercise can raise the body's core temperature to dangerous levels that risk fetal health, especially during the first three months of pregnancy.

Warning Signs that Indicate the Need to Stop Exercising

If you have any of the following symptoms while you're exercising, stop immediately and contact your doctor or midwife.

- pain for more than a moment anywhere, but especially in your back or pelvic region
- excessive fatigue during or following exercise
- dizziness during or following exercise
- shortness of breath during or following exercise
- feeling faint during or following exercise
- vaginal bleeding
- difficulty walking
- abdominal contractions
- absence of fetal movements over a reasonable time period

You should also discontinue your exercise program and contact your health care provider if you have a rapid heartbeat during exercise and/or while resting.

Modifications to an Aerobic Exercise Program

Important modifications to the traditional aerobics class need to be made for pregnant women. The following is a list of general modifications and guidelines adapted from both the American College of Obstetricians and Gynecologists (ACOG) and a symposium, lecture, and video course called *Pregnancy the Aerobic Way*, developed by Bonnie Rote, RN and AFAA consultant, and Kenneth Sekine, MD.

Warm-Up

The warm-up should be longer than in regular classes, due to the pregnant woman's increased risk of orthopedic

Altered body alignment: Pregnant versus non-pregnant

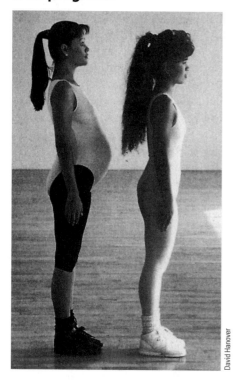

David Hanover

injury. Ten to twelve minutes is the minimum time period suggested for warm-up. During pregnancy, estrogen and progesterone cause tissues and joints to soften and become unstable. When joints are unstable, ligaments and tendons are in greater danger of tears or strains. The enlarged breasts and uterus alter the center of gravity and produce a greater strain on the lower back. An increased load is also placed on the sacroiliac and hip joints, which can feel like a sore tailbone at times.

It is fatiguing for pregnant exercisers to maintain proper body alignment while standing; therefore, many thoughtful teachers have developed methods of warming up while on the floor. Smooth, controlled, static stretches are essential to a proper warm-up. Static stretches for the hamstring, inner thigh, and calf can all be performed on the floor. Ballistic movements should never be performed during warm-up or cool-down.

Rhythmic limbering is the second essential element to a proper warm-up. Mild walking and rhythmic upper body movement are both good warm-up exercises.

Cardiovascular Work

During pregnancy, the mother's blood volume increases by 50 percent. This dilute volume results in a lower oxygen-carrying capacity, which reduces the cardiac reserve during physical activity. In addition, the expanding uterus reduces the size of the lung cavity, causing a mild hyperventilation during rest that does not increase proportionately with exercise. Overall, this means that many pregnant women may be unable to maintain high levels of aerobic activity.

To adapt to aerobic work when pregnant, lower your target heart rate to 60 percent of the maximum for beginners, gradually increasing to 70 percent of the maximum for intermediate-to-advanced exercisers. It's wise to maintain a target heart rate of 65 percent during the final stages of pregnancy. The American College of Obstetricians and Gynecologists recommends never

exceeding 140 beats per minute (see the target heart rate calculations).

The amount of time spent in continuous aerobic movement should not exceed 15 minutes, according to ACOG. Use how you feel as a guideline for workout. A useful measure is Borg's Perceived Exertion Scale, since the heart rate response itself may be variable and inconsistent.

The following chart is adapted from Swedish physiologist Gunnar Borg. Select a number within this range that best describes your level of exertion, and multiply that number by 10. The resulting product may be close to your working heart rate.

Floor Work

The floor work portion of the class is important to the pregnant participant. A greater portion of the prenatal class is dedicated to floor work because: (1) the exercises performed during floor work can directly relate to relaxation exercises for labor; (2) the time spent on gentle stretching and toning exercises can relieve much of the discomfort of pregnancy; and (3) floor work provides a stable base of support for exercise.

Abdominal exercises should not include any strain or feeling of "bearing down," which may occur in regular classes. The rectus abdominis muscle often has a normal midline separation during pregnancy. It's important to guard against further separation of this muscle by only doing modified abdominal work on your hands and knees. Abdominal work should never be performed at a fast pace or with a sudden, jerky movement. A pelvic tilt, with the lower back pressed

Borg's Scale of Perceived Exertion	
20	Very, very hard
18	Very hard
16	Hard
14	Somewhat hard
12	Moderate
10	Light
8	Very light
6	Very, very light

Inner and outer thigh work: Side leg lifts

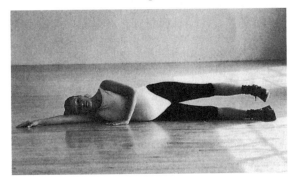

a.

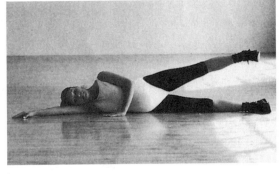

b.

Abdominal curls with arm variation

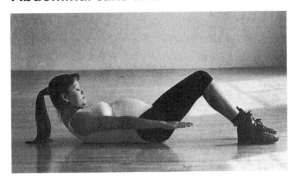

a. Arms at hips

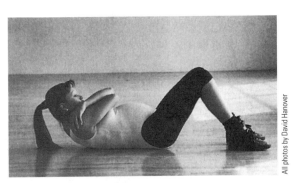

b. Arms crossed over chest

All photos by David Hanover

to the floor, should be maintained throughout abdominal curls.

A good alternative to abdominal curls is to get on all fours and gently pull the abdomen in and contract while exhaling. Make sure the back does not arch.

In advanced pregnancy, modify the abdominal work so that you roll back from an upright-seated position to a backward lean of only 45 degrees. However, this movement primarily works the hip flexors, and the abdominals run a distant second.

Exercises for the back of the thigh should be reduced in number and intensity, if not eliminated. These exercises include extending and lifting the leg while in an all-fours position. The weight of the abdomen stresses the lower back when leg lifts are performed. Increased pressure on the diaphragm

makes breathing difficult, and added strain is placed on the small, round ligaments near the groin.

Perform both inner and outer thigh work in the side-lying position, lying all the way down rather than up on your elbow. This keeps the spine in better alignment.

Cool-Down Stretches

Perform as many stretches on the floor as possible. In this way, you get the maximum support for your unstable posture. Instead of taking static stretches to the point of maximum resistance, do slow, controlled, relaxing stretches.

Make sure your heart rate is well below 60 percent of your maximum heart rate before getting on the floor for your final floor work and cool-down stretches.

Alternative to abdominal curls

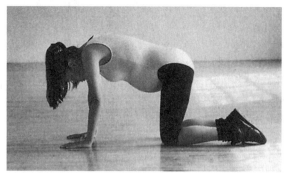

a. Contracting the abdomen

b. Extending the back

Floor work: Gentle limbering stretch

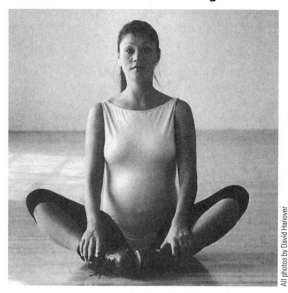

All photos by David Hanover

Special Exercises

Low-Impact Movement

Low-impact or aqua aerobics classes are definitely the way to go during pregnancy. Caution should be given to exaggerated upper body movement. Refrain from lifting the arms so high that the back arches and the abdomen protrudes even further.

Kegel Exercises

Muscles of the pelvic floor are not usually exercised in a regular aerobics class. Responsible for supporting the pelvic organs, these muscles hold the uterus floor in place and can prevent urinary incontinence and sexual dissatisfaction. Kegel exercises strengthen these muscles, located between the pubic bone in front and the coccyx in back, which should be emphasized in a pregnancy class. You can do these "invisible" little exercises by imagining the area at the base of your pubic region is like an elevator floor. When you contract the right muscles, the elevator floor rises a few inches. These are the same muscles you use when you try to stop the flow of urine.

During pelvic tilts, use Kegel exercises to strengthen these muscles. These Kegel exercises should be done both early in the pregnancy and throughout a woman's lifetime.

Standing Work

It is recommended that you warm up the lower back, midback, shoulders, and upper back before making any lateral, side-bending motions. A gentle head drop and forward shoulder roll can loosen tension in the upper body and back.

Standing waist work should be performed at half the speed of the regular repetitions. Never lean so far to the side that you lose your balance. Also, doing a stretch to one side with both arms overhead (double overhead arm side stretches) should never be done. Always lift upward, with only a slight side bend when warming up the side muscles.

Upper bodywork for muscular endurance can be safely performed in a standing position as long as special attention is paid to proper body alignment: knees should be soft, never locked; feet should be shoulder-width apart; toes pointing out slightly; hips tucked under slightly; rib cage lifted; abdominals held in to support the lower back; shoulders back and down; and head held high.

Controversial Exercises

Whether pregnant women should exercise on their backs is one of the most controversial issues in exercise and pregnancy. ACOG does not recommend exercises from a back position after the fourth month of pregnancy. Many physicians and other programs, including *Pregnancy the Aerobic Way (PAW)*, disagree, reporting that many women sleep on their backs, and labor on their backs, without incident.

If you are pregnant and lying on your back, your blood vessels may be compressed, leading to a fall in blood pressure, dizziness, and fainting for you, and decreased oxygen for the fetus. If these symptoms arise, avoid back-lying exercises. If back-lying positions do not create a problem, *PAW* recommends that exercises under 3 minutes in length be performed. Roll to your side for a rest period before proceeding to the next exercise.

Exercises to Avoid

High Knee Lifts

High knee lifts create an irritation and soreness in the round ligaments that run diagonally down the sides of the pelvis and suspend the uterus in the pelvic cavity.

Quick Lateral Movements

Rapidly shifting direction with quick lateral movements can increase the chance of falling, since your center of gravity is thrown off balance. Overly rapid lateral movements can also put a torque motion on the knees, causing strain and injury.

High-Impact Jumping and Jarring

High-impact movements are not recommended if you are pregnant. The increased weight adds to orthopedic injuries of the lower back, hips, knees, shins, ankles, and feet. Your altered center of gravity also increases the risk of falling during jumping. Instead, turn a heel-jack or jump-kick into a step-with-heel-out.

Weights

The use of wrist or ankle weights during pregnancy is not recommended. If pregnant, you are fully challenged by adjusting to the addition of 15 to 35 extra pounds. You need no further workload added to your already taxed musculoskeletal framework.

Traditional Rejects

Basically, the same exercises that lead to injury in a regular aerobics class should be avoided if you are pregnant. These include plough, hurdler's stretch, full neck circles, standing toe touches, deep knee bends, double leg lifts, straight leg sit-ups, kneeling donkey kicks, deep leg lunges, and inverted bicycling. Most importantly, avoid all forward flexion unless your upper body weight is well-supported.

Prone Position

Any prone (lying on the stomach) exercises are too uncomfortable and dangerous. Push-ups fall in this category.

Summary

1. In general, as long as a pregnant woman is in good health and has medical clearance from her physician, she can safely participate in a low-impact aerobics class.

2. Prenatal exercise classes should be taught by trained professionals who are prepared to meet the physical and emotional needs of the pregnant exerciser.

3. Some important modifications can make the aerobics class a safe, enjoyable experience.

4. Warm-ups are often extended so that the changing orthopedic structure of the pregnant woman is adequately prepared. Both rhythmic limbering and mild walking are good warm-up exercises.

5. During cardiovascular work, the pregnant exerciser is cautioned against reaching heart rate exceeding 140 beats per minute, or 80 percent of her maximum heart rate.

6. During floor work, part of the class may be devoted to relaxation exercises that help prepare for labor.

7. Alternatives to abdominal curls are important so that any normal separation of the rectus abdominis is not at risk in advanced stages of pregnancy.

8. Certain exercises, such as Kegel exercises, lower back stretches, and gentle groin stretches, can alleviate much of the discomfort of pregnancy and add to the importance of a prenatal class.

9. Exercises that irritate and stress the supporting ligaments should be avoided.

10. Safety is the key factor for pregnant exercisers. An aerobics class should not only be safely modified, but should incorporate special exercises and adaptations to assure strength, endurance, flexibility, and well-being for both mother and fetus.

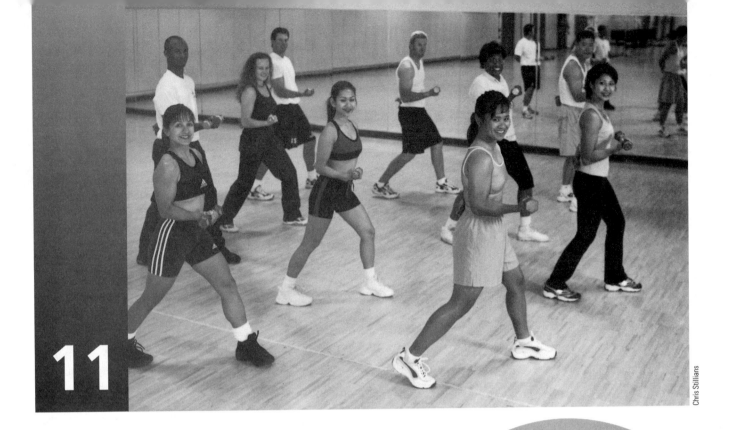

Chris Stillians

11

Selecting a Class

Outline

What to Look for in a Good
    Instructor
Characteristics of a Good
    Instructor

The Aerobic Dance Exercise Class
Checklist for Selecting a Facility
Selecting a Facility
Summary

What to Look for in a Good Instructor

When you think about signing up for a dance exercise class, you may wonder where to begin. There are many teachers to choose from and many places to take classes. Some people erroneously think that if the instructor looks good, then that person must be a good instructor. Unfortunately, many establishments employ instructors based on their appearances instead of their qualifications. After reading this chapter, you will know the right questions to ask to seek out a qualified instructor. If you take classes from a qualified instructor, you will be able to get the most out of your workout.

Characteristics of a Good Instructor

Good instructors teach with enthusiasm and genuine concern for their students. They come to class well-prepared to teach, and arrive in ample time to set up the room and begin on time. An instructor should always start a class promptly and finish on time. Before the series of classes begins, a good instructor explains the goals of aerobics, how and why to take your pulse, and how to determine your target heart range. A good aerobics instructor should be a role model, a person who is fit, and someone who lives a healthy lifestyle. This does not mean that your instructor should look like he or she walked off the cover of a magazine—not all good instructors look like movie stars. Other very important characteristics of a good instructor are that he or she has a professional affiliation with an educational resource organization and demonstrates a commitment to continuing education. Your instructor should have a fitness certificate or an equivalent certification from a university or a private certifying organization.

It is very important for your safety that your instructor shows a knowledge of the appropriate applications of exercise physiology and injury prevention by demonstrating only safe and effective exercise techniques. Also, your instructor should be able to modify the exercises for those with special needs, such as the overweight or pregnant exerciser. Another very important certification that your instructor should have is cardiopulmonary resuscitation (CPR).

Does the instructor conduct the class in a nonintimidating and noncompetitive manner? That's how a good class should be conducted. Is he or she there for a personal workout or for YOU? Is the instructor conscious of how the environment is affecting the class? Is it too hot or too cold? Is the music too loud? Are people bumping into one another? A good instructor will be cognizant of these factors and make the appropriate adjustments. The instructor should be aware of the fatigue level of the class and look for signs of overexertion. Similarly, individuals who do not appear to be working hard enough might need additional encouragement.

The Aerobic Dance Exercise Class

Every instructor has a unique style, and that's good! However, all classes should follow the same basic formula. First, there should be a 7- to 10-minute warm-up that includes all major muscle groups and avoids ballistic stretches. Following the warm-up will be the aerobic section of the class, which lasts for 15 to 30 minutes, depending on the overall length of the class. During this time, there should be a gradual build-up, a sustained high-intensity level, and a gradual decrease in intensity. Finally, it is important to have the post-aerobics cool-down, where intensity gradually decreases so as not to shock the system with a sudden change of pace. Your instructor should guide you in checking your pulse rate 5 minutes into the aerobics class, as well as at the end of the aerobic section. There should also be a post-aerobic recovery check 2 to 3 minutes after cool-down.

Checklist for Selecting a Facility

1. Is it conveniently located?
2. Are there classes given at the times you desire?
3. What is the composition of the aerobics floor? Is it shock absorbent?
4. Are there weight-training facilities?
5. What are the qualifications of the instructors for aerobics and for weight training?
6. Are there other facilities, such as weights or a swimming pool?
7. What social activities are offered (socials, dances, trips, tournaments)?
8. Can you afford the membership fee?

The organization of the dance exercises should flow smoothly and skillfully from one movement to another and one section of class to the other. The cues given by the instructor should be easily understood, and the movements should be challenging and keep your interest. Too much time spent on one activity without variation leads to boredom. A good instructor changes the movements frequently, yet allows enough repetition so you can eventually be successful.

A good class also includes about 15 minutes of exercises to strengthen the muscles of the arms, chest, shoulders, abdomen, back, legs, buttocks, and hips. A 5-minute cool-down includes static stretches for every muscle group worked.

Selecting a Facility

A good facility or club makes you feel good about yourself and makes you want to return to work out again. A well-run facility is concerned about your welfare, not just your membership. A qualified, concerned director hires only qualified instructors and makes sure they are familiar with the equipment and safety skills. A good facility maintains a clean, hygienic environment. The showers, restrooms, and locker rooms are clean and well-maintained. The temperature is well-regulated in the workout and dressing areas. A good facility has a suspended or coiled-wood floor, high-density matting, or absorbent flooring material in the aerobics room.

If the facility has weight equipment, the area should be effectively supervised with qualified leaders. The equipment should be well maintained and in good working order. Policies should be established and enforced to allow all members easy accessibility to the equipment. A facility with weight training equipment should be set up so you can keep a log of your progress and file it in the workout area for easy accessibility each time you exercise.

When selecting the facility, be sure to check the schedule of classes. Does it offer classes at times you can attend? If it doesn't, the facility won't be of much use to you. Does it demonstrate a willingness to adapt to the clients' requests for different time slots, more classes, and a variety of offerings; for example, low-impact, prenatal, and high-impact? Are other services available, such as a nutritionist, physical therapy, massage, and a referral network of physicians in case of injury? Is the facility convenient to your home or work? Does it provide childcare facilities? Does the membership fee fit into your budget?

All of these considerations should be well-evaluated when selecting a facility. Select the facility that best meets your needs. If you don't, you may find you have joined a club you won't really use. So take time to investigate the facility before you join. It will save you money and aggravation in the future.

Summary

1. Your most important consideration in selecting a workout facility is the instructor you choose for your class. A good instructor:

   - is certified by an accredited organization and/or is university trained
   - holds a CPR (cardiopulmonary resuscitation) card
   - arrives on time and begins on time
   - is clear and thorough about the goals of the class
   - acts professionally
   - gives feedback to students
   - assists you in finding your target heart rate
   - conducts the class in a nonintimidating manner

2. Characteristics of an effective class:

   - 7 to 10 minutes of warm-up
   - 15 to 30 minutes of aerobic work that keeps you at your target heart rate
   - 3 to 5 minutes of aerobic cool-down
   - Approximately 15 minutes of strength development and toning
   - 5 minutes of cool-down activities and flexibility

3. A facility should have:

   - a soft floor (suspended or coiled-wood floor), absorbent flooring, or mats
   - clean and well-maintained areas
   - classes at convenient times
   - friendly, helpful staff members

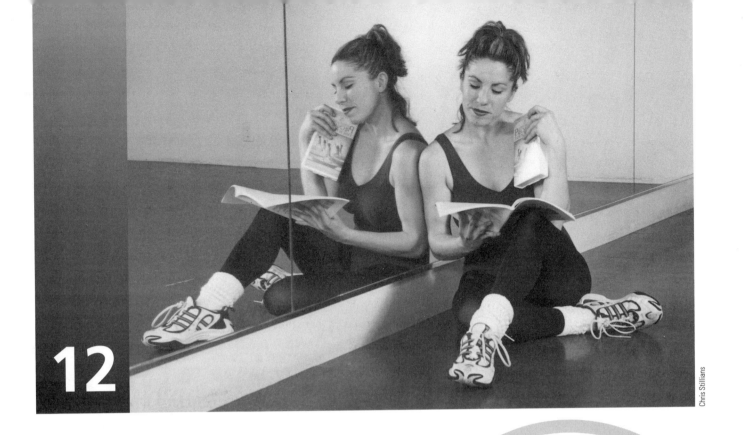

12

A Guide to Buying Media for Personal Use

Outline

Selecting a Videotape
Evaluating a Videotape
Purchasing a Videotape
Selecting Music to Create Your
    Own Routines

Checklist: Videotape Evaluation
Summary

You may find that you occasionally have to miss an exercise class and you'll need to work out at home or in a motel room while you are traveling. To prepare for that situation, you can buy a videotape (for home use) or music (to use at home or when traveling) to motivate you through your own routine. Here are some guidelines for buying your media.

Selecting a Videotape

There are over 150 aerobics videotapes on the market from which to choose. The videotapes vary in ability level and style. However, for the most part, these home video workouts attempt to offer you a safe, effective, informative exercise program that you can execute at any location. Some videos simply present the exercise material, others give you extensive scenery and elaborate camera angles. Before you purchase a videotape, preview it or rent it so you can evaluate whether it meets your needs.

Evaluating a Videotape

In evaluating a videotape for purchase, rate the following five areas as they relate to your needs: instructor technique, balance and flow of the class, safety, technical proficiency of the production, and the overall effectiveness of the videotape for your purposes.

Purchasing a Videotape

With such a wide selection of videotapes available, it is highly probable that your local vendor doesn't carry all of them. First, investigate what tapes your local vendor carries, and find out whether you can preview them, or at least rent them. Check out the supply at another vendor and again see whether you can preview the tapes of your choice. Use the previous Checklist for Evaluation to help you make your selection. Since you will be using the tape more than once, it is important that it meets your needs and that you are satisfied with it before you purchase it. A catalog is available that describes most of the exercise tapes on the market. It may be worth sending for it before you purchase a videotape. To order your free cat-

alog, send your name and address to:

> Video Exercise Catalog
> Department AR7
> 5390 Main Street NE
> Minneapolis, MN 55421

Videotapes are also available from bookstores, variety stores, and from:

> Aerobics and Fitness Association of America
> 15250 Ventura Blvd.
> Suite 200
> Sherman Oaks, CA 91403

Selecting Music to Create Your Own Routines

When creating your own routines, you need to decide what music to use. The simplest solution, of course, is to use music you already have. However, the tempo won't necessarily be appropriate for the exercises you want to do. You can spend hours attempting to find the right music.

A number of companies sell music for aerobics, in which they have adjusted the tempo of contemporary songs to fit warm-up, aerobics, strength and flexibility exercises, and cool-down. Here are several of the companies from which you can order music for aerobics; additional companies can be found with an Internet search:

> Dance Tracks
> 91 East Third Street
> New York, NY 10003

> Music In Motion®
> Headquarters in Ithaca, New York
> Phone: 607-257-6196 or Tollfree
> 877-646-3262 (877-MIM-DANCE)
> East Coast Music Productions, Inc.
> P. O. Box 3812
> Gaithersburg, MD 20878

> Musicflex
> 159-34 90th Street
> Queens, NY 11414

> Dynamix Music Service, Inc.
> 9411 Philadelphia Road
> Baltimore, MD 21237

Checklist Videotape Evaluation

After viewing the videotape, check the *yes* or *no* column for each question. Once you have completed the checklist, add up your *yes* responses and your *no* responses. If you have significantly more *yes* responses, the videotape is acceptable.

Instructor Technique   Yes   No

1. Does the instructor give adequate cues to guide you into the movement?

2. Can you follow the choreography?

3. Do you like the choreography?

4. Are the transitions smooth?

Class Balance   Yes   No

1. Does the class include all five parts of a good lesson: warm-up, aerobics, aerobic cool-down, strength and flexibility, and an overall cool-down?

2. Is the time allotted to each section of the class properly balanced?

    warm-up: 7 to 10 minutes

    aerobics: 15 to 30 minutes

    aerobic cool-down: 5 minutes

    strengthening and toning: 15 minutes

    overall cool-down and flexibility: 5 minutes

3. Is the entire body worked out in the routine?

Safety Information   Yes   No

1. Does the instructor discuss proper body alignment and or proper ways to execute each exercise?

2. Are the demonstrations executed with proper body alignment?

3. Is there an accompanying guide book that discusses exercise precautions?

4. Is time allotted to check your target heart rate?

Technical Proficiency   Yes   No

1. Are the camera angles appropriate for you to understand the movement?

2. Do the camera angles assist your learning or detract from it?

3. Is it difficult to follow the movement because of the way it is photographed?

4. Is the music well-recorded?

5. Do you like the music?

6. Is the cuing properly coordinated with the demonstration?

Overall Effectiveness   Yes   No

1. Does the videotape provide you with a model you can follow?

2. Is the videotape presentation of the class motivating to you?

3. Did you enjoy exercising to the tape?

4. Did the tape provide you with the workout you need?

    Total number of *yes* responses_____

    Total number of *no* responses_____

    Did you have more *yes* responses than *no* responses?

After evaluating a videotape, review the checklist. If the responses are mostly positive, the tape should work for you. If the responses are mostly negative, keep reviewing videotapes until you find one that meets your needs.

Summary

1. Sometimes it is difficult for you to attend a dance exercise class, so you may want to have an aerobics videotape to follow on your own time.

2. Before you purchase a videotape, evaluate it for quality and suitability.

3. There are more than 150 videotapes on the market for exercising at home or when you are traveling.

4. You may want to purchase recorded music to perform your personal workout to when you are traveling or when you can't get to class.

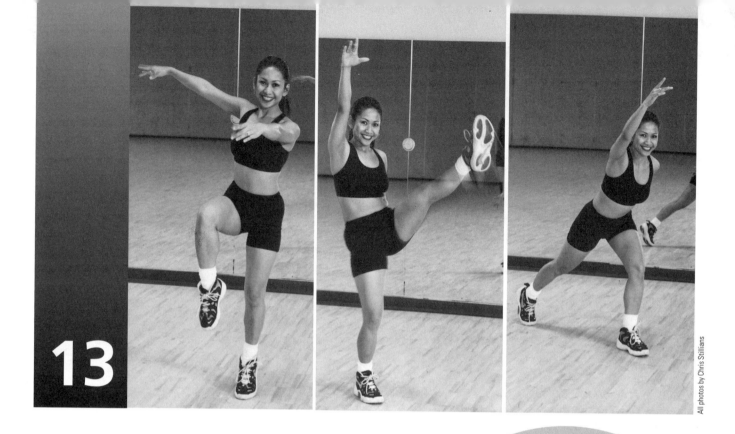

13

Being Creative: Choreographing Your Own Routines

Outline

Creating Your Dance Exercise
    Routine

Simple 8-Count Phrases of
    Movement
Summary

Many students like to create (choreograph) their own dance exercise routines to music they enjoy. Choreographing your own routines can be a very creative and satisfying experience. Before you begin, remember that the goal of aerobic dance exercise is to combine dance steps and movement patterns, coordinated with music, that keep you moving continuously so you can exercise your body and heart. The workout should be 15 to 30 minutes long, allowing you to reach your target heart rate and receive the exercise training effect you desire. If you want high-impact routines, use movements that have a lot of bounce. If you want low-impact routines, keep one foot in contact with the floor at all times. You can also create routines that combine high- and low-impact activities. This type of a routine offers you variety and gives you a good workout.

Creating Your Dance Exercise Routine

First, select your music. The music should have a steady beat as well as a motivating "upbeat" feeling that makes you want to work hard. There are many sources for buying pre-recorded music appropriate for routines. Once you select your music, listen to it and analyze the musical phrasing. Usually, the music is composed such that you can create phrases of movement that take 8 counts. You can create several phrases of 8 counts of movement, and then combine them in various ways to "fit" the composition of the music. Each phrase you create can be given a letter to identify it. If you create 4 phrases, letter them A, B, C, and D. Then combine the phrases in any order you like; for example, A B C D A B A B C D. The phrases can be repeated in any order, and as many times as you desire, as long as they fit with the music. Another variation that you can use is repeating the one phrase 4 times, making it a 32-count phrase, and changing the direction of the movement on each repetition.

A

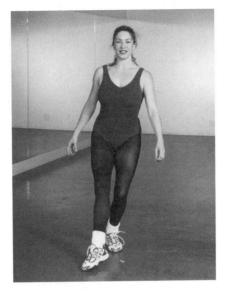
a. Hop and point front

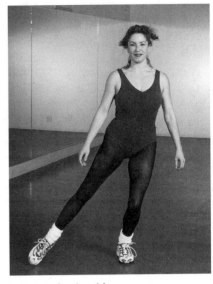
b. Hop and point side

B

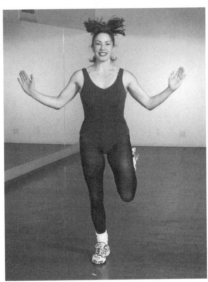
a. Run and clap

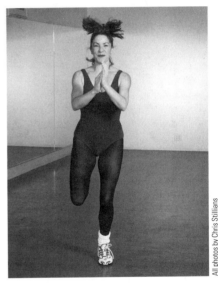
b.

All photos by Chris Stillians

You don't have to be a dancer to create an enjoyable, high-energy routine. An example of 4 phrases of movement (identified as A, B, C, and D) that you could combine into a routine is:

A: Hop on the left foot 4 times while pointing and tapping the right foot forward, and then to the side (for example, forward, side, forward, feet together on count 4, jump/change sides). Repeat the entire phrase while hopping (bouncing) on the right foot 4 times and tapping the left foot forward and to the side as described. Repeat the phrase again on each side.

B: Run in place 8 times, clap on each run.

D

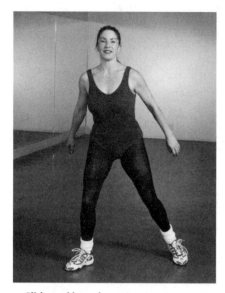

a. Slide and hop clap

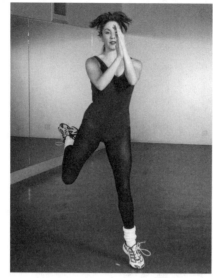

b.

Walking in place

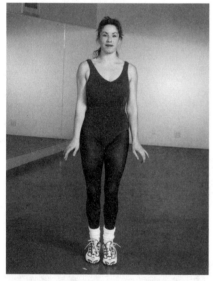

a. Arm variations

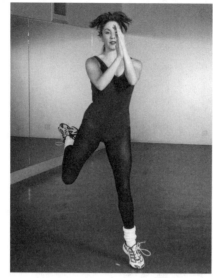

b.

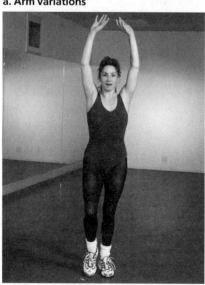

c.

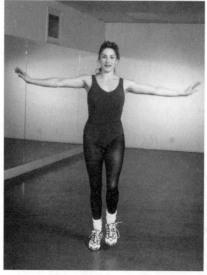

d.

C: Do 8 jumping jacks, using full arm movements.

D: Slide to the right 8 times, clap on the eighth slide. Repeat to the left.

These phrases can be first performed in the A B C D format, and then combined in any order you feel works well with the movement. A simple way to add variety is to do different arm movements each time you repeat the phrase. When you make a variation, identify that lettered phrase with a subscript number. For example, let's say the original phrase is lettered "A." The next time you repeat "A," but vary the arm movements, identify the phrase as "A_1." Your new routine might be: A B C D A_1 B_1 C_1 D_1 A B C D.

In this routine, you use the original 4 phrases, change the arm movements that accompany each phrase, then repeat the original 4 phrases of movement.

A more challenging and diversified routine has more than 4 phrases to combine. It is up to you how many phrases you would like to create and use in each routine. Movement phrases longer than 8 counts may be difficult for you to remember at the beginning. However, when you become more experienced, you can challenge yourself and create longer routines and utilize more complex movements.

The phrases you use in your dance exercise routines are only limited by your abilities and creativity. So, have fun and create the routines to which you would like to exercise!

You can use the following 8-count phrases of movement in any order in creating your own dance exercise routines, or combine them into 32-counts. These are only representative of the types of steps you can use; there is really no limit to the phrases you can create. Be creative and have fun!

Simple 8-Count Phrases of Movement

■ Jump in place 8 times while hitting the sides of your thighs with straight arms.

■ Walk in place on your toes, performing 16 steps while moving your arms

Mountain Climber

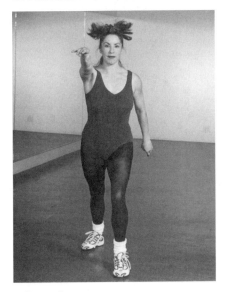

a. Front view

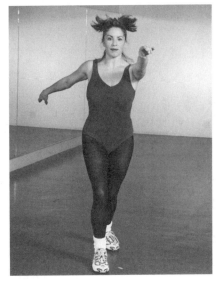

b. Alternating feet

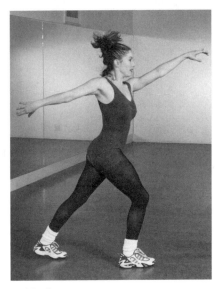

c. Side view

Pony

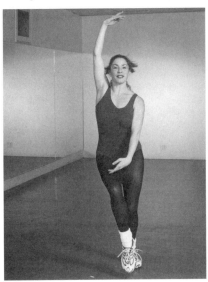

a. Hop, step, step

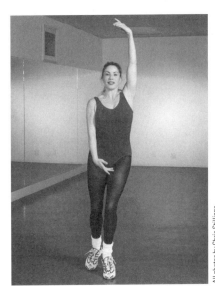

b. Other side

All photos by Chris Stillians

down and up on the sides or in front of your body.

■ Run in place 8 times while lifting your feet high in the rear.

■ Run in place 8 times while lifting your knees high in front.

■ Perform 8 jumping jacks, moving your arms down and up in coordination with the leg movements.

■ Perform 8 jumping jacks, moving your arms down and only half way up (to the shoulder level) in coordination with each leg movement.

■ *Mountain Climber:* With your feet separated, jump and land forward and backward a distance of about one foot. Alternate feet as you land in front and in back on each jump. Your arms can swing high in opposition to the leg movements.

■ *Pony:* "Hop, step, step." Hop on the right foot to the side, and then quickly step with the left foot and then the right foot. Repeat on the other side.

■ *Heel, toe, slide, slide:* Hop on the left foot while tapping the right heel to the

Heel Toe Slide

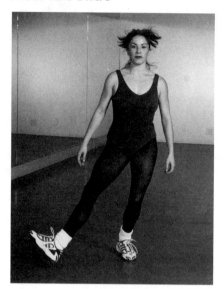

a. Hop, heel side

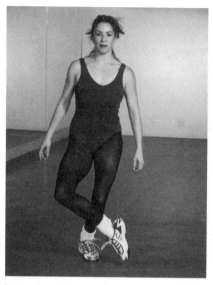

b. Hop, cross toe

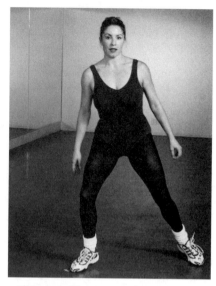

c. Slide and slide

Hop Swing

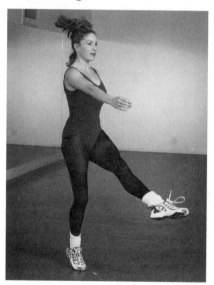

a. Alternate legs

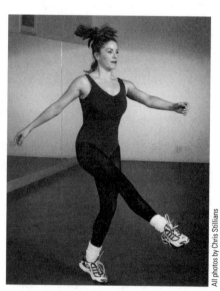

b.

right side. While hopping again on the left foot, swing the right foot to the front and touch the toe on the floor. Perform two slides to the right. Repeat the entire phrase by hopping on the right foot and sliding to the left.

■ Hop on one foot and lift up the opposite knee. Reverse.

■ Hop on one foot, and swing kick the opposite foot forward. Reverse.

■ *Charleston Bounce Step:* Use a very bouncy step throughout this phrase.

Step right, kick the left foot forward, step back on the left foot, and touch the right toe back. Repeat 8 times. Reverse.

■ *Can-Can Kick:* Hop on the right foot, and simultaneously bring the bent left knee up high in front. Hop again on the right foot, lightly touch the left foot on the floor next to the right, and kick the left foot into the air. Repeat 4 times, and then repeat on the other side. A more advanced version involves alternating sides after each kick.

Hop, slide

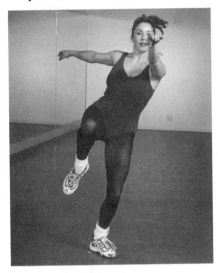

a.

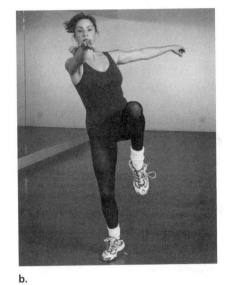

b.

Charleston Kick

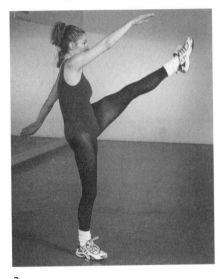

a.

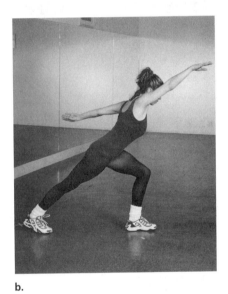

b.

Can Can Kick

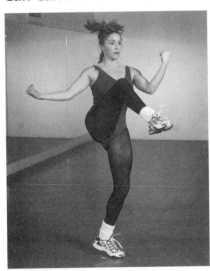

a. Pull arms down

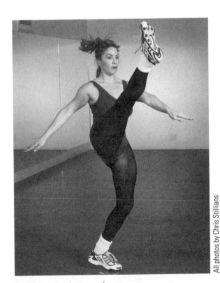

b. Then, swing and press arms

Grapevine

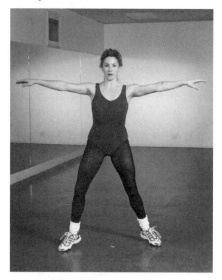

a. Step side

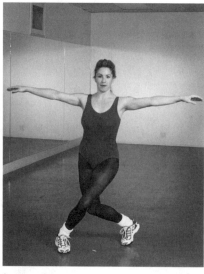

b. Cross front

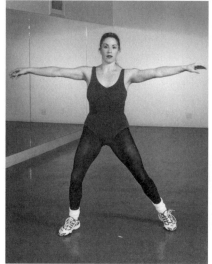

c. Step side

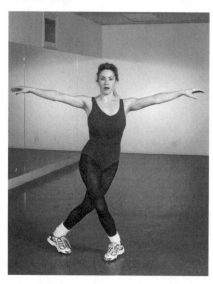

d. Cross back

Grapevine Schottische

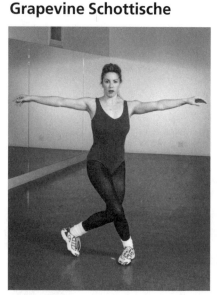

a. Cross front

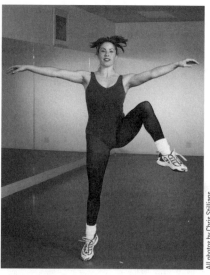

b. Step side

c. Hop

- *Schottische:* Run 3 times in place or while traveling, and hop and clap simultaneously (Run R, L, R, hop R). Alternate sides 4 times.

- *Grapevine:* While traveling to the right, cross the left foot over the right, step to the right on the right foot, cross the left foot behind the right, and step on the right foot while traveling to the right. Repeat this phrase 4 times, moving to the right. To perform the grapevine in reverse with a smooth transition, begin by stepping on the left foot to the left before crossing the right foot over the left.

- *Grapevine schottische:* Step to the right on the right foot, cross the left foot behind the right, step on the right to the right, and hop on the right. To reverse, step on the left foot to the left, cross the right foot behind the left, step on the left foot to the left, and hop on the left foot. Repeat 4 times.

- Run 3 times in place, and kick and clap on the 4th count. Alternate sides. Repeat the phrase 4 times.

- Twist the body while using a bounce landing, and swing the arms in opposition overhead on each twist. The arms can also be swung from side-to-side at chest level.

- *Jump kick:* Jump and kick the right foot forward, then jump and kick the left foot forward. Vary the movement by kicking the leg on a diagonal and alternating the

All photos by Chris Stillians

Twisting the Body

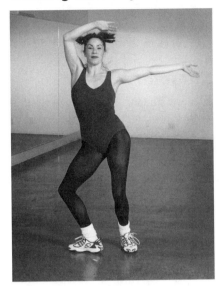

a. Arms swing overhead

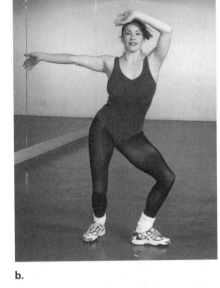

b.

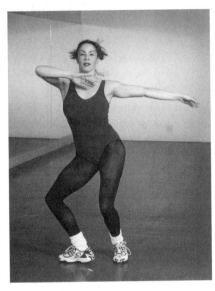

c. Arms swing center

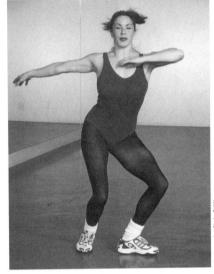

d.

direction of the kick. Perform 8 jump kicks, alternating sides.

■ *Skiers' jump:* Jump to the right while twisting the body toward the left diagonal. Reverse on the other side. Perform 8 times. For variety, you can jump twice on each side before changing directions.

■ Run forward R, L, R, hop on the R foot while lifting the L knee and L arm up; run backward (reversing the movement) L, R, L, hop on the L foot while lifting the R knee and R arm up. For variety, you can add a pivot turn on the hop and change directions.

■ For a low-impact variation, complete the phrase described above without hopping on the last movement. Instead, lift up to the ball of your foot.

Jump Kick

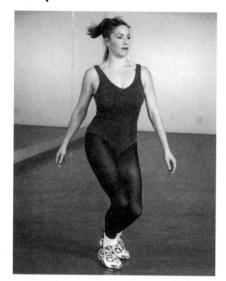

a. Jump

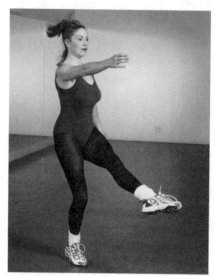

b. Kick

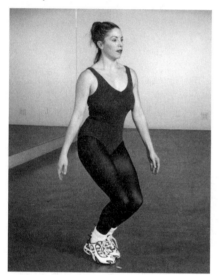

c. Jump

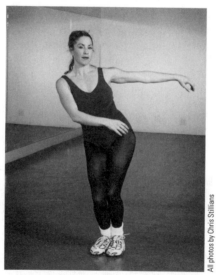

d. Kick opposite foot

Skiers Jump

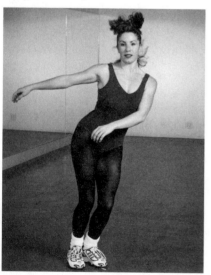

a.

b.

Summary

1. Many students like to choreograph their own routines. They find it a creative experience to create routines to music they enjoy.

2. The aerobic routine you create should last 15 to 30 minutes and be strenuous enough to allow you to reach your target heart rate.

3. Select music that motivates you and has a steady beat.

4. Create movement phrases consisting of 8 counts each. Label each phrase with a letter, such as A, B, C, and D. Then combine the lettered phrases the way they best fit the music; for example, A B C D A C D D B A. There is no limit to the way you can combine your movements. Have fun!

5. You can combine 4 phrases of 8-count movements and identify it as a 32-count phrase if you would like.

6. Remember to monitor your heart rate every 5 minutes to see whether you are staying in your target heart rate zone.

All photos by Chris Stillians

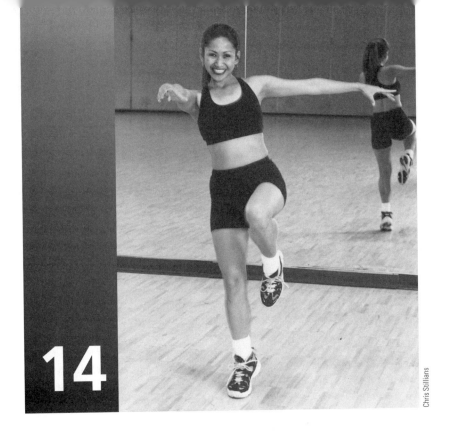

Chris Stillians

14

Becoming an Instructor

Outline

Where to Study to Become an
    Instructor
Checklist: Do I Want to Become
    an Instructor?

Summary
Self-Test

Many dance exercise participants who have taken classes for a long period of time begin to wonder if they might enjoy teaching aerobic dance exercise classes themselves. The purpose of this chapter is to provide you with the answer to the question: *What do I have to do to become an aerobic dance exercise instructor?* To become an aerobic dance exercise instructor, one must first enjoy the activity of aerobic dance exercise. Secondly, an aerobic dance exercise instructor must be in top physical condition. Third, persons interested in teaching aerobic dance exercise must study exercise physiology, anatomy and kinesiology, nutrition and weight control, components of teaching aerobic dance exercise, first aid, and cardiopulmonary resuscitation. Finally, one interested in teaching aerobic dance exercise must enjoy working with and helping people.

There is a movement in this country to require all aerobic dance exercise instructors to be certified. However, at this point, there is no such national mandate. The certification requirement rests with each individual state or private business manager. At present, no state requires dance exercise instructors to be certified either within their state or with a nationally recognized certification. Many universities offer fitness instructor certificates that are recognized by hiring agencies. Many employers are requiring their instructors to be certified. That is a good sign of a quality, well-run organization.

Consumers deserve to be taught by the very best person available to teach a dance exercise class. If a class is taught by an individual that is good looking, but uneducated, the participants run the risk of being injured, and the organization runs the risk of a liability lawsuit. Today's dance exercise participant is an educated consumer. Participants will stop attending a class taught by an uneducated individual. It is to the agency's advantage to hire well-trained instructors. Hence, if you would like to become an instructor, you will need to start taking classes and studying.

Where to Study to Become an Instructor

One of the first places to investigate procedures for becoming an instructor is at your local university or college. Many universities and colleges offer fitness instructor certificates. If you study at a university, you can trust that well-educated, knowledgeable instructors are teaching you. If your local university does not provide a certificate, then your next source is a private agency. There are over 50 private organizations offering fitness instructor certificates or dance exercise instructor certificates. The quantity and quality of instruction varies greatly from one organization to the next. You must thoroughly investigate the various courses you will be studying and the time spent in each course. In investigating the curriculum, be sure to see that there are course offerings in the following subjects:

- exercise physiology
- anatomy and kinesiology
- nutrition and weight control
- components of teaching aerobic dance exercise
- health screening, and modifying for individual variations
- first aid
- cardiopulmonary resuscitation

Since there are over 50 private organizations certifying individuals in the teaching of aerobic dance exercise, it is very confusing to decide if you should become certified, with which organization to become certified, or if you should become certified by a university. The decision is yours. You must study the options available to you.

The six largest and most recognized certifications are offered through:

The Aerobics and Fitness
Association of America
15250 Ventura Boulevard, Suite 310
Sherman Oaks, CA 91403
Phone: (818) 905-0040

Checklist:
Do I Want to Become an Instructor?

1. Am I interested in leading and help-ing other people exercise?
2. Am I good at motivating people?
3. Am I well-liked?
4. Can I express myself well?
5. Do I have the desire, time, and money to go to school to study to be-come an instructor?

6. Am I a good role model for an in-structor of dance/aerobic exercise?
7. Am I willing to study for the courses necessary to become an instructor?

If you answered *yes* to these questions, you might make a good instructor. Per-haps it is time for you to investigate the local schools and/or organizations that certify dance exercise instructors.

American College of Sports
Medicine
P.O. Box 1440
Indianapolis, IN 40206
Phone: (317) 637-9200

American Council on Exercise
5820 Oberlin Drive, Suite 102
San Diego, CA 92121-3787
Phone: (858) 535-8227 or
(800) 825-3636
Fax: (858) 535-1778

National Dance Exercise Instructor
Training Association
5955 Golden Valley Rd, Suite 240
Minneapolis, MN 55422

Y.M.C.A.
101 N. Walker Drive
Chicago, IL 60606
Phone: (312) 269-0516
IDEA (*a provider of continuing
education for instructors*)
6190 Cornerstone Court E, Suite 204
San Diego, CA 92121
Phone: (800) 999-4332

If you do decide to become an aerobic dance instructor, it is imperative that you take courses in the subjects previously mentioned! You want to do the best job you can as an instructor. To do that, you must be well-qualified and educated in all of the aspects of teaching aerobic dance exercise. Good luck to you!

Summary

1. To become an aerobic dance exercise instructor, you must enjoy aerobic dance exercise and motivating other people.

2. You need to be in top physical condi-tion to be an aerobic dance exercise instructor.

3. You must study many subjects so you will be well-prepared to be the best instructor you possibly can. The sub-jects you will need to study are: phys-iology, anatomy and kinesiology, nutrition and weight control, compo-nents of teaching aerobic dance exer-cise, first aid, and cardiopulmonary resuscitation.

4. Investigate the various places where you can study to become an instructor. They are at universities and private agencies and are listed in the chapter.

5. Good luck to you, and happy studying!

Self-Test

1. List two personal characteristics an individual must possess to become an aerobic dance exercise instructor.

_____

_____

_____

2. To become an instructor, one must study the following courses:

   exercise physiology

   anatomy and kinesiology

   nutrition and weight control

   components of teaching aerobic dance exercise

   first aid and cardiopulmonary resuscitation

   Write the subjects listed above that you have already studied.

   _____

   _____

   Write the subjects you are most interested in learning more about.

   _____

   _____

   List the subjects you are least interested in.

   _____

   _____

3. Aerobic dance exercise instructors must be certified to teach in the United States. True or false?

4. Many employers require their instructors to be certified. True or false?

5. List two places at which you can study to become a certified aerobic dance exercise instructor.

   _____

   _____

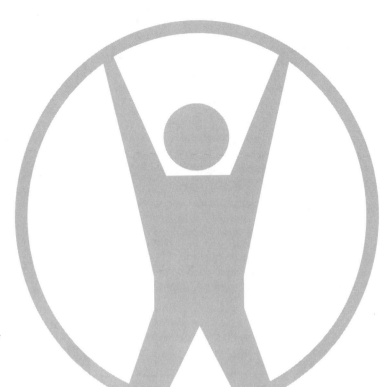

Glossary

Abduction is moving a body segment (such as an arm or leg) away from the center of the body (such as raising one's arms from the side to the side at shoulder height).

Adduction is bringing the body segment back to the center of the body (such as bringing arms back from an abducted position).

Aerobic refers to the use of oxygen during exercise.

Aerobic capacity (cardiorespiratory endurance) is the ability of the body to remove oxygen from the air and transfer it through the lungs and blood to the working muscles.

Aerobic dance exercise is a form of movement and exercise that incorporates a variety of dance movements performed at various tempos to motivating music.

Aerobics is a popular form of exercise that incorporates vigorous, bouncy locomotor movements to provide a fun form of fitness development and exercise.

Agonist is a muscle contracting concentrically, such as the biceps in a curl.

Alignment refers to the correct positioning of the spine and the body parts. Alignment has postural implications referring to how all the body parts line up.

Amino acids are the building blocks of protein; organic compounds containing nitrogen, hydrogen, and carbon.

Anaerobic means without oxygen; usually referring to short spurt, high-energy activities such as sprinting.

Arteriosclerosis is a general term for a disease that leads to the thickening and hardening of the inner layer of the artery wall due to fat deposits. It causes a decrease in the inner diameter of the artery.

Artery is the large blood vessel that carries oxygenated blood away from the heart to the body tissues.

Ballistic movements are jerky, bouncy, explosive, and unsustained movements.

Basal metabolic rate is the sum total of energy required by all the physiologic processes required to maintain life; the number of calories burned to sustain life.

Blood pooling refers to a condition caused by ceasing vigorous exercise too abruptly so that blood remains in the extremities and may not be delivered quickly enough to the heart and brain.

Blood pressure refers to the amount of pressure the blood exerts against the walls of the arteries during each heart contraction and heart relaxation. Taking the blood pressure measures the pressure of the blood in the arteries.

Body alignment refers to how the torso, limbs, spine, shoulders, head, etc. are positioned. Proper body alignment refers to the optimal placement and posture of the body during exercise to ensure safe, injury-free movement.

Body composition is the proportion of body fat to lean body mass (muscle, bone, cartilage, and vital organs). Proper body composition is a part of overall fitness.

Calorie is the common word used to refer to the kilocalorie. A kilocalorie is a measure of the value of foods that produce heat and energy in the body. One calorie is equal to the amount of heat required to raise the temperature of one gram of water one degree Centigrade.

Carbohydrate refers to organic compounds containing carbon, hydrogen, and oxygen; when broken down, carbohydrates are the main energy source for muscular work and one of the basic foodstuffs in the diet.

Cardiovascular efficiency refers to the ability of the body to deliver oxygen to all of its vital organs efficiently during the stress of exercise.

Carotid pulse is the pulse located on the carotid artery just under the jawbone. It is the common area used for taking the heart rate during and following exercise, as it is quickly and easily located.

Cholesterol is a chemical compound found in animal fats and oils. High levels of cholesterol in the blood are often associated with a high risk of arteriosclerosis.

Chronic refers to something persisting over a long period of time.

Coronary arteries are the two main arteries arising from the aorta and arching down over the top of the heart. They are the major arteries responsible for carrying blood to the heart muscle.

Diastolic pressure is blood pressure within the arteries when the heart is in relaxation between contractions.

Duration is the length of time devoted to an exercise or an exercise session.

Ectomorph is a body type or somatotype. This type of a person appears thin, lean, and has a delicate bone structure.

Empty calories refer to food which yields calories that are void or nearly void of nutrients, protein, vitamins, and minerals. This usually involves foods containing high sugar content, fat content, and alcoholic beverages.

Endomorph is a body type or somatotype. This type of a person appears soft and round with a predominance of fat tissue, but is not necessarily obese.

Extension is increasing the angle of a joint (such as straightening your arms from a bent position).

Fat is stored in the body as adipose tissue. It serves as a concentrated source of energy for muscular work; a compound containing glycerol and fatty acids.

Fatigue refers to a diminished capacity for work as a result of prolonged or excessive exertion.

Flexibility is the range of motion in the joints.

High-impact refers to a form of aerobics that incorporates jumping and bouncing movements. There is a high degree of impact placed on the joints, bones, and feet in this form of aerobics class.

Hyper-extension is when the angle of a joint is moved past the normal range of motion.

Intensity is the level of difficulty of an exercise or a workout.

Lordosis refers to an increased lumbar curve or a "sway back".

Low-impact refers to a form of aerobics that keeps one foot on the floor at all times; aerobics classes that involve no jumping.

Low-intensity refers to a reduced workload, or working at a lower target heart rate.

Mesomorph is a somatotype or body type describing the very muscular, athletic looking individual.

Metabolism is the chemical reaction of a cell or living tissue that transfers usable materials into energy.

Muscular endurance is the ability of the muscles to exert force over an extended period of time.

Muscular strength is the amount of force produced when a muscle group contracts and moves a resistance.

Nautilus is a type of weight machine which uses special cams to change the amount of force needed to lift the weight so that the muscle will be working closer to maximum throughout the exercise.

Overload is the method used to increase the workload beyond the normal capacity to improve and develop muscular strength and endurance.

Overuse syndrome refers to nagging ailments that result from exercising too much, too soon; these can involve muscles, tendons or bones, and respond to a treatment of rest, ice, compression and elevation.

Perceived exertion refers to a means of measuring how hard one is exercising by comparing a subjective self-rating with an established chart of various levels.

Prone means lying face down.

Radial artery is the artery that is located on the inside of the wrist. It lies very close to the surface of the skin and is therefore often used for counting the pulse.

Recovery heart rate is how quickly your pulse returns to normal after an aerobic workout.

Repetition is one complete action of an exercise.

Resting heart rate refers to the number of times your heart beats per minute when you have been sitting or resting for approximately 10 minutes.

RICE is the acronym for rest, ice, compress, and elevate: the steps for immediate injury treatment.

Risk factors are genetic and non-genetic characteristics which contribute to the incidence of heart disease or stroke.

Set point theory proposes that human metabolism works very hard to maintain a certain body weight; that weight is held in place through complex homeostatic mechanisms.

Shin splints is a catch-all phrase used to describe any discomfort in the front of the lower leg; usually a result of overuse syndrome.

Side stitch refers to a pain in the side during exercise. It is thought to be caused by a spasm in the diaphragm, due to insufficient oxygen supply and improper breathing.

Sprain is a wrenching or twisting of a joint in which ligaments are stretched past their normal limits.

Static stretching movements place the muscle in a sustained stretch position for a given period of time. This is an effective way to achieve flexibility in a specific muscle group. It is the opposite of ballistic stretching movements.

Strain is a "muscle pull"; a stretch, or a tear of the muscle or adjacent tissue.

Strength is the maximum force or tension that a muscle or muscle group can produce against a resistance.

Supine means lying face up.

Target heart rate is the level at which you will gain the benefits of exercising your heart to improve cardiovascular fitness.

Tendon is a band of dense fibrous tissue forming the termination of a muscle, which attaches muscle to bone with a minimum of elasticity.

Tendonitis is an inflammation of a tendon; often requires several weeks of rest to completely heal.

Time refers to the length of time devoted to a workout, a class, or a particular exercise.

Training effects are the physiologic adaptations that occur as a result of aerobic exercise of sufficient intensity, frequency, and duration to produce beneficial changes in the body.

Triglycerides are compounds composed of glycerol fatty acids. They are stored in the body and are unhealthy when stored in high levels.

Vein is a blood vessel carrying blood away from the body and toward the heart.

Vertebrae are the bony or cartilaginous segments, separated by discs, that make up the spinal column.

Warm-up is a balanced combination of static stretch and rhythmic limbering exercises that are used to prepare the body for more vigorous exercise.

Working heart rate is the heart rate taken at the completion of the aerobic section of the workout to identify if the individual was in his or her target heart rate zone and at the proper intensity for his or her age and physical fitness level.

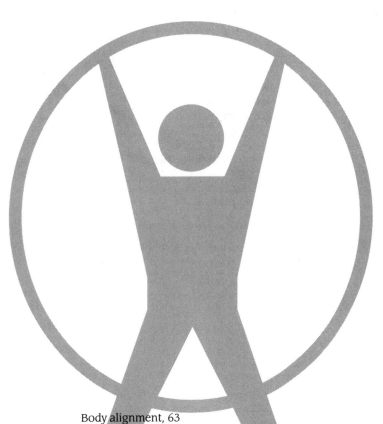

Index

Abdominal curl-ups, 46–48
Achilles' tendonitis, 61
Aerobic capacity, 34–36
Aerobics class
    cardiovascular/aerobics work, 22
    cool-down and flexibility, 23
    strengthening and toning work, 23
    warm-up and stretching, 21, 22
Aerobics
    benefits, 7, 21, 29
    defined, 2
    how much to do, 4, 5, 12, 13
    mental benefits, 29
Alcohol, 18
Anatomical diagrams, 64, 65
Ankle circles, 44, 45
Ankle raises, 44, 45
Aqua Aerobics Today (Casten), 74
Aqua exercise, 73, 74
Asthma, 68
Aversion therapy, 27

Back arching, 66
Bad cholesterol, 17
Bad exercises (exercises to avoid),
    63–68, 81
Ballistic stretching, 22, 63
Basal metabolic rate (BMR), 55
Becoming an instructor, 99–102
Bent side leg lifts, 49, 50
Blair, Steven, 4
Blood cholesterol level, 17
Blood pressure, 17
BMI, 15, 16
BMR, 55

Body alignment, 63
Body composition, 8, 56
Body mass index (BMI), 15, 16
Body sculpting, 2
Body shape, 14
Body types, 8, 9
Body weight, 14–16
Borg, Gunnar, 78
Borg's scale of perceived exertion, 78
Bouncing stretches, 22, 63
Brown fat, 55

Calf stretches, 44
Calorie/weight chart, 16
Can-can kick, 94, 95
Carbohydrates, 53
Cardiovascular disease
    prevention, 19
    risk factors, 13–18, 69
    symptoms, 68, 69
Cardiovascular efficiency, 8
Cardiovascular endurance, 8
Catecholamine, 7, 74
Charleston bounce step, 94, 95
Checklists
    becoming an instructor, 101
    desirable body weight, 56
    first aerobics class, 22
    food groups, 54
    knee protection, 72
    mental benefits of aerobics, 29
    mental imagery, 31
    personal goal setting, 30
    personal workout, 51
    selecting a facility, 85

Checklists—*continued*
  semester progress chart, 39
  taking the pulse, 10
  treating injuries, 60
  videotape evaluation, 89
  warm-up, 23
Cholesterol, 14, 17
Choreographing your own routine,
  90–98
Chrondomalacia, 61
Cigarette smoking, 14
Clothes, 24
Cooper, Kenneth, 4
Core board training, 3, 4
Coronary heart disease, 14
Creating your routine, 90–98
Cross trainer shoes, 24

Deep lunge, 43
Diabetes, 18
Diet. *See* Nutrition
Dietary guidelines, 56, 57
Donkey leg lifts, 48
Drinking water, 67
Duration of exercise, 13

Ectomorphic body types, 8, 9
8-count phrases of movement, 92, 93
Endomorphic body types, 8, 9
Endorphins, 21
Excess body weight, 14
Exercise buddy, 31
Exercise intolerance, 68
Exercises to avoid, 63–68, 81

Fats, 54
Fiber, 53
Fitness assessment, 32–39
Fitness awareness, 13
Flexibility, 8
Flexibility testing, 31, 37
Food. *See* Nutrition
Food groups, 53, 54
Food guide pyramid, 57
Frequency exercise, 12
Frequency of workouts, 23, 24
Full sit-ups, 67

Goals, 29, 30
Good cholesterol, 17
Grapevine, 96
Grapevine schottische, 96

Hamburger, Marc, 3
Hamstring stretch, 43, 44
Hand-held weights, 72, 73
HDL, 17
Head isolations, 41
Health history, 37, 38
Healthy People 2010, 4

Heart attack, 14
Heart disease. *See* Cardiovascular
  disease
Heart rate, 9–12
Heat, 67
Heel toe slide, 94
Heel walking, 45
High blood cholesterol, 17
High blood pressure, 16, 17
High-density lipoprotein (HDL), 17
Hip circles, 42
Hip isolations, 42
Hop swing, 94
How much to do, 4, 5, 12, 13
Humidity, 67
Hurdler's stretch, 66
Hydration, 54
Hyperextension, 66
Hypertension, 16

Ideal body weight, 14, 15
Imagery, 30
Incentive therapy, 27
Injury prevention, 59–69
  cardiac risk factors, 69
  causes of injury, 62, 63
  exercise intolerance, 68, 69
  exercise-induced asthma, 68
  exercises to avoid, 63–68
  heat/humidity, 67
  high-impact movements, 71
  knee protection, 72
  low-back precautions, 72
  overuse injuries, 61
  pain vs. exercise discomfort, 60
  RICE, 60, 61
Inner-directed people, 28
Instructor, 84
Instructor certification, 100, 101
Intensity of exercise, 12

Jump kick, 96–98

Karvonen method, 11
Katz, Jane, 73
Kegel exercises, 80
Kick boxing, 2
Knee injuries, 61, 62
Knee protection, 72

LDL, 17, 18
Louganis, Greg, 30
Low-back precautions, 72
Low-density lipoprotein (LDL), 17, 18
Low-impact aerobics, 70–75
  aqua exercise, 73, 74
  benefits, 74, 75
  body sculpting, 74
  defined, 71

other low-impact alternatives, 74
   weights, 72, 73
Low-intensity, 73

McKechnie, Alex, 3
Measurements, 33–35
Mental benefits, 29
Mental visualization, 30
Mesomorphic body types, 8, 9
Motivation, 26–31
Mountain climber, 93
Muscle groups, 63
Muscle imbalance, 63
Muscular endurance, 8
Muscular strength, 8
Music, 88

Negative motivation, 27
Nutrition, 52–58
   body composition, 56
   dietary guidelines, 56, 57
   food groups, 53, 54
   vitamins and minerals, 54, 55
   water/hydration, 54
   weight control, 55
   weight loss, 56

Outer-directed individuals, 28
Overuse injuries, 61

Pelvic lifts/buttocks exercises, 50
Personal goals, 29, 30
Personal measurements, 33–35
Physical inactivity, 18
Pilates, 2, 3
Pilates, Joseph H., 2
Plantar fasciitis, 61
Pony, 93
Positive motivation, 27, 28
Pre-class warm-up, 41
Pregnancy, 76–82
   cardiovascular work, 78
   controversial exercises, 81
   cool-down stretches, 79
   exercises to avoid, 81
   floor work, 78, 79
   Kegel exercises, 80
   low-impact movement, 80
   special precautions, 77
   standing work, 80
   warm-up, 77, 78
   warning signs, 77
Progress log, 31
Proteins, 53, 54
Pulse, 9, 10
Push-ups, 45–47

Quadriceps stretch, 44

Recovery heart rate, 12
Reverse push-ups, 46, 47
Rib circles, 42
Rib isolations, 42
RICE, 60
RISKO factor profile, 58
Rockport fitness walking test, 11
Runner's high, 29

Schottische, 96
Selecting a class, 83–86
Selecting a facility, 84, 85
Self-motivated people, 28
Semester progress chart, 39
Set-point theory, 55
Shin splints, 61
Shoes, 24, 25
Shoulder circles, 42
Side leg lifts, 48, 49
Side leg swings, 68
Side lunge, 43
Side to side twisting, 68
Sit-and-reach test, 36, 37
Sit-ups, 67
Sitting straddle forward stretch,
   45, 46
Sitting straddle side stretch, 45, 46
Skier's jump, 97, 98
Smoking, 14
Somatotypes, 8, 9
Sorensen, Jacki, 2
Spinning classes, 2
Sprained arch, 61
Static stretches, 22
Step aerobics classes, 2
Straight leg lifts, 48, 49, 66
Strengthening exercises, 45–50
Stress, 18
Stress fractures, 61
Stress reactions, 61
Stretching
   ballistic, 22, 63
   static, 22
   types of exercise, 41–45
Stroke, 14
Sweat, 54

Taking the pulse, 9, 10
Target heart rate, 10–12
Testing your fitness level, 32–39
TH, 7
Thomi, Manuela P., 3
3-minute step test, 34–36
Training heart rates chart, 34
Twisting the body, 97
Tyrosine hydroxylase (TH), 7

Videotape, 88, 89
Visualization, 30
Vitamins and minerals, 54, 55

Waist circumference, 16
Walking in place, 92
Warm-up, 21–23, 41
Water, 54, 67
Water aerobics, 73, 74
Weight control, 55

Weight loss, 56
Weights, 72, 73
Windmill toe touches, 67
Wrist weights, 72

Yoga plough, 66